Life-Threatening Cardiac Emergencies for the Small Animal Practitioner

The *Rapid Reference* Series

Books in the *Rapid Reference* series are ideal quick references, using a concise, practical approach to provide small animal practitioners with fast access to essential information. Designed to be used at a patient's side, these books make it easy to quickly diagnose and treat patients. With a spiral binding to lie flat, *Rapid Reference* books are an indispensable tool for the exam room.

Life-Threatening Cardiac Emergencies for the Small Animal Practitioner

Maureen McMichael DVM

Diplomate American College of Veterinary Emergency and Critical Care
Professor
College of Veterinary Medicine
University of Illinois
Urbana, Illinois

Ryan Fries DVM

Diplomate American College of Veterinary Internal Medicine (Cardiology)
Clinical Assistant Professor
College of Veterinary Medicine
University of Illinois
Urbana, Illinois

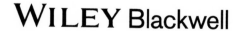

This edition first published 2016 © 2016 by John Wiley & Sons, Inc.

Editorial offices: 1606 Golden Aspen Drive, Suites 103 and 104, Ames, Iowa 50010, USA

The Atrium, Southern Gate, Chichester, West Sussex, PO19 8SQ, UK

9600 Garsington Road, Oxford, OX4 2DQ, UK

For details of our global editorial offices, for customer services and for information about how to apply for permission to reuse the copyright material in this book please see our website at www.wiley.com/wiley-blackwell.

Library of Congress Cataloging-in-Publication Data

Names: McMichael, Maureen, author. | Fries, Ryan, author.
Title: Life-threatening cardiac emergencies for the small animal practitioner/
    Maureen McMichael, Ryan Fries.
Other titles: Rapid reference.
Description: Ames, Iowa : John Wiley & Sons, Inc., 2016. | Series: Rapid
    reference series | Includes index.
Identifiers: LCCN 2016015883 (print) | LCCN 2016019412 (ebook) | ISBN
9781119042075 (paper) | ISBN 9781119042099 (pdf) | ISBN 9781119042082
    (epub)
Subjects: | MESH: Heart Diseases–veterinary. | Emergencies–veterinary. |
    Pets.
Classification: LCC SF811 .M36 2016 (print) | LCC SF811 (ebook) | NLM SF 811
    | DDC 636.089/612025–dc23
LC record available at https://lccn.loc.gov/2016015883

A catalogue record for this book is available from the British Library.

To my mother, Ann. You taught me so much. I love you and miss you every day.

M.M.

To Katie for her love and support. To my parents for helping me achieve my dreams.

R.F.

Contents

Preface

One of the most frightening emergency presentations for veterinarians is that of a pet with a life-threatening cardiac condition. A cat with dull mentation and a heart rate of 110 bpm is a critical emergency as is the dog with a heart rate of 300 bpm. The diagnosis and treatment of these animals cannot wait and in many cases treatment must be instituted before a final diagnosis is reached. Our goal with this book is to create a clear, up-to-date practical guide to help veterinarians streamline the process of treating emergent cardiac patients. This book emphasizes the clinical approach in order to facilitate a rapid diagnosis or, in some cases, treatment before the diagnosis is made. The book is filled with numerous ECG images, thoracic radiographs, and echocardiogram images accompanied by clear, concise directives for emergency treatment.

The book is separated into five sections to streamline identification: Bradyarrhythmias, Tachyarrhythmias, Miscellaneous arrhythmias and cardiac conditions, Electrolyte disturbance and the ECG, and Algorithms and drug chart. With a total of six chapters, four algorithms, and a drug chart, all common life-threatening cardiac arrhythmias that occur in small animals are covered. Additionally, in the "Miscellaneous arrhythmias and cardiac conditions" section, we have added six emergency conditions that are frequently associated with arrhythmias: Congestive heart failure from mitral regurgitation in dogs, congestive heart failure from cardiomyopathy in cats, cardiogenic shock from dilated cardiomyopathy in dogs, arteriothromboembolism in cats, caval syndrome from heartworm disease in dogs, and pericardial effusion in dogs. These were added to give practitioners step-by-step guidance on how to treat the non-arrhythmia aspects of these life-threatening emergencies.

This is a hands-on manual, very low on theory, and it is meant to be used cage side. This book is meant for students (to streamline the material they are learning), veterinarians in training, and veterinarians in practice who need a quick source that enables rapid diagnosis and treatment in the face of a pet with a dangerous cardiac arrhythmia or cardiac emergency.

We know how frightening emergent cardiac conditions can be and we aim to empower veterinarians with the answers in a quick and easy-to-use format. Then, after the animal is stabilized, the theory and pathophysiology of cardiovascular disease can be read in depth in a comfy chair by the fire. There are several excellent textbooks on cardiovascular disease suggested in the "Further reading" section.

Good luck out there,

Kind regards,
Maureen and Ryan

Acknowledgments

We would like to thank our teachers and mentors who have given us the foundation to begin learning. We thank all of the wonderful technicians we have worked with, without them we would fall apart. We also thank our colleagues and referring veterinarians who keep us on our toes and push us to learn more every day. Our residents are a constant source of inspiration, showing us what can be achieved and pushing past us on this amazing road of knowledge. We thank all of the interns and students we have worked with who show us an unending curiosity and excitement for the material; without it, we might forget what an amazing profession this is. We thank Wiley-Blackwell for their vision and support throughout this project. Most importantly, we thank our clients for trusting us with their precious pets, which teach us every day what unconditional love really is.

Acknowledgments

We would like to thank our teachers and instructors who have given us the foundation to begin learning. Without all of our wonderful teachers we have worked while without them we would fall apart. We also thank our colleagues and students who keep us on our toes and push us to learn more every day. Our students are a constant source of inspiration, showing us what can be achieved and pushing past it in the amazing field of knowledge. We thank all of the interns and students we have worked with who show us an amazing enthusiasm and excitement for the material without which we might have went an amazing profession there. We thank Wiley-Blackwell for their vision and support throughout this project. Most importantly, we thank our clients for trusting us with their precious pets, which reminds us every day just how rewarding our job really is.

Introduction

Life-threatening arrhythmias and cardiac conditions can be very intimidating to diagnose and treat. This book is meant to provide a concise guide to the rapid diagnosis and treatment of arrhythmias in dogs and cats, as well as a resource for the most common life-threatening cardiac conditions. We start with the normal ECG and this chapter is designed for re-familiarizing the practitioner with the basics of ECG recording and evaluating. The book is then split into sections based on the heart rate. Bradyarrhythmia and tachyarrhythmia sections are followed by miscellaneous arrhythmias and cardiac conditions. This organization has been structured to allow the practitioner to evaluate the rate first, go to the accompanying section, and find a match for the arrhythmia. Additional life-threatening cardiac conditions that may or may not be associated with an arrhythmia can be found under the "Miscellaneous arrhythmia and cardiac conditions" section. The algorithms are meant as a quick guide to arrhythmia detection and treatment and the drug chart has up-to-date cardiac medications along with commonly used drug dosages in dogs and cats.

Chapter 1 Normal ECG

This chapter serves as a brief overview of how to perform an ECG, what it measures, and what a normal ECG looks like. We hope to provide a baseline of understanding that will put the rest of the book into context and set the stage for optimal ECG recording and diagnosis. Practitioners familiar with the basics of ECG recording and interpreting may wish to skip this chapter.

Before recording

Before beginning the ECG a physical examination (either a complete physical if the animal is stable or a triage physical) is performed. A triage physical exam is focused on life-threatening body systems (heart, lungs, mentation) while putting the additional non-life threatening aspects of the physical exam off until the animal is stable (e.g., rectal exam, fundic exam, and so on). Listening to the heart and lungs, feeling the pulses, evaluating perfusion (mentation, pulse strength, mucous membrane color, body temperature, etc.) are all essential components of evaluating a cardiac arrhythmia.

The stethoscope has a bell (the smaller side on a two-sided stethoscope), which picks up low frequency sounds. On a stethoscope with only one side the bell picks up low-frequency sounds with gentle pressure against the thorax. Low-frequency sounds are best for detecting a gallop rhythm (heart sounds 3 and 4). The diaphragm (larger side on a two-sided stethoscope) picks up higher frequency sounds, including murmurs and clicks. In a stethoscope with only one side the diaphragm picks up high-frequency sounds with more firm pressure against the thorax. The ear pieces are inserted into the ears facing forward and stethoscopes with smaller diaphragms (pediatric and neonate) are essential for practitioners who examine small-sized (puppy, kitten) and exotic patients.

Life-Threatening Cardiac Emergencies for the Small Animal Practitioner, First Edition. Maureen McMichael and Ryan Fries.
© 2016 John Wiley & Sons, Inc. Published 2016 by John Wiley & Sons, Inc.

ECG set up

The pet is placed in right lateral recumbency on a pad or towel if they are stable. Padding the table minimizes electrical interference from the metal table. A cold table without padding may also increase artifact by causing the animal to shiver or keep changing positions in an attempt to get more comfortable. If the animal is not stable they should be allowed to remain in whatever position is most comfortable while recording the ECG.

One person should hold the animal with limbs extended (forelimbs extended toward the head and rear limbs extended toward the tail) and 70% isopropyl alcohol should be placed between the ECG clips and the animal to increase contact. When a signal is either unclear or absent additional alcohol can be added and it may need to be re-applied frequently. The traumatic alligator clips hurt (try them) and atraumatic clips (which are flat and do not pinch) should be used whenever possible. These may decrease resistance (and artifact) on the part of the animal as they are significantly more comfortable. Adhesive electrodes are best for long-term use.

Minimizing sounds and movement are essential for proper interpretation of the ECG. Respiratory sounds (holding the mouth closed in a panting, but stable animal), shivering (towel or pad under the animal), or purring (turning on tap water) should all be eliminated or minimized to the extent possible while always keeping the animal's health status uppermost in mind.

The clips are placed with the white lead (RA; right arm) on the right forelimb near the back of the triceps, the black lead (LA; left arm) on the left forelimb near the back of the triceps, the red lead (LL; left leg) on the left rear limb just proximal to the stifle on the front of the thigh, and the green lead (RL; right leg, grounding lead), if used, on the right rear limb just proximal to the stifle on the front of the thigh.

Recording the ECG

Leads allow an assessment of the electrical activity of the heart from several different angles. Each angle is called a lead. The standard ECG includes all six of the limb leads; lead I, II, III, aVR, aVL, aVF. Generally a rhythm strip is produced at the bottom of the page and is most often a longer run of lead II.

Paper speed is very important and ideally two different speeds should be used for assessment. A recording for 30–60 s, at 25 mm/s is done first. This slower speed allows more complexes on the strip and helps to assess for abnormalities in the rhythm (e.g., ventricular premature contractions, atrial premature contractions, and so on). This is followed by recording of a rhythm strip (usually lead II) at 50 mm/s for 2–3 min or longer depending on the disorder.

The standardization signal should, ideally, be set at 1 cm = 1 mV, which means that each tiny square equals 0.1 mV in height. If this standardization is changed the complexes may look very small or very tall and a misdiagnosis can occur.

What is measured

Electrical impulses move through the heart via the specialized conduction system starting at the sinoatrial node, moving to the atrioventricular node and then down the bundle of His to the Purkinje fibers. In a normal heart the muscle contracts in response to this electrical stimulus. It is important to note that the ECG only records the electrical activity of the heart and does not assess contractility. The echocardiogram is the gold standard for cardiac function and chamber enlargement. We recommend a new book in this series, *Echocardiography for the SA practitioner*, by June Boon. It is a concise manual of performing and interpreting echocardiograms in small animals.

Normal ECG

The P wave represents atrial depolarization and P waves can be positive (upright), negative (downward), or biphasic. The QRS complex represents ventricular depolarization.

The Q wave is the first negative deflection following the P wave and it is followed by the R wave. The R wave is the first positive deflection after the P wave (the Q wave may not be present or visible). R waves should always be positive in lead I. The leads should be checked for position on the patient if this is not the case. The S wave is the negative deflection that follows the R wave. The T wave represents ventricular repolarization (relaxation) and T waves can be positive (upright), negative (downward), or biphasic. Not all of these waves must be present in an ECG but every R wave must be followed by a T wave. This is helpful when trying to decide which wave is present between two R waves—if there is truly only one it must be a T wave.

Calculating the heart rate

There are several ways to calculate the heart rate. We will only describe two here. More can be found in resources in the "Further reading" section. The number of R-R intervals between two sets of marks can be counted. These are the tick marks at the top of the ECG paper. This equates to 3 seconds if the paper speed is 50 mm/s. This number (the number of R-R intervals between the tick marks) is then multiplied by 20 to get the heart rate. Alternatively an average-sized pen

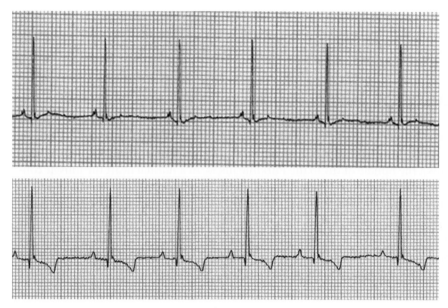

Figures 1 and 2 Normal ECG Canine.

can be placed on the strip and the R-R intervals counted between one end of the pen and the other. This number can be multiplied by 20 (if the paper speed is 50 mm/s). If the paper speed is 25 mm/s the number of R-R intervals between tick marks (or using the pen) can be multiplied by 10 "pen times ten." Always verify the heart rate on the ECG machine or that calculated by the above methods, with auscultation of the animal.

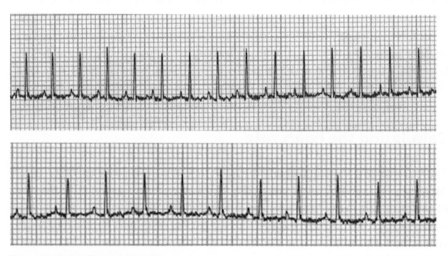

Figures 3 and 4 Normal ECG feline.

Calculating the mean electrical axis

The mean electrical axis (MEA) reflects the area of the heart that takes the longest for electrical depolarization to travel through. In normal hearts it is the left ventricle (the thickest part of the heart muscle). If there is hypertrophy of the right ventricle the MEA may shift to the right. It may also be shifted if there is a conduction disturbance (i.e., bundle branch block), which slows down the ventricular depolarization in the area of the block. The normal MEA for dogs is +40 to +100 degrees and for cats it is −5 to +160 degrees. There are several ways to calculate the MEA (see "Further reading" for excellent cardiology texts) and for the sake of brevity we will describe only one here. An isoelectric lead is one where the complexes have an equal amount of positive and negative deflection so that the total electrical energy is net neutral. It is usually the smallest complex seen on the ECG. If an isoelectric lead can be identified then the MEA is perpendicular to that lead. For example, if the isoelectric lead is aVL then the MEA is aVR, which is either +30 degrees or −150 degrees. If the QRS is positive in aVR then the MEA is +30, whereas if the QRS is negative in aVR then the MEA is −150.

Measuring the complexes

The height of the P wave is measured from baseline to the top of the P wave. The width of the P wave is measured from the inside of the start of the P wave to the end of the P wave. An increase in either height or width, or both, may point to atrial enlargement. An increase in height may point to right atrial enlargement and is called P-pulmonale. An increase in P wave width may indicate left atrial enlargement and is called P-mitrale. Notching of the P wave may also be an indicator of left atrial enlargement. An absent P wave may be either artifact (check all leads) or may be seen with atrial fibrillation, junctional rhythms, and some other arrhythmias. Normal values for dogs and cats can be found in references in the "Further reading" section.

The P-R interval is measured next and is measured from the beginning of the P wave to the beginning of the Q wave. It reflects AV junction activation and prolongation suggests that the impulse is slowed down traveling through the AV node (first-degree heart block).

The width of the QRS complex is measured from the beginning of the Q wave to the end of the S wave (where it comes back to baseline). There are nuances that may make measurement here difficult (e.g., no Q wave etc.) and the "Further reading" section has a wealth of information for those interested in delving more deeply into ECGs. The height of the R wave is measured from the baseline (where it starts) to the top of the R wave and the depth of the Q or S wave is measured from baseline to the deepest part of the respective wave. Increased duration of the QRS suggests abnormal ventricular depolarization (e.g., left bundle branch block) and increased height of the R wave suggests left ventricular enlargement. A small amplitude R wave may indicate pericardial effusion, severe pleural effusion, and hypothyroidism. The S wave, when increased in height (i.e., deeply negative) suggests right ventricular enlargement while increases in width suggest abnormal depolarization of the right ventricle (e.g., right bundle branch block).

The ST segment is measured from the baseline at the end of the S wave (i.e., where it returns to baseline) to the beginning of the T wave and represents early ventricular repolarization. Elevation may indicate myocardial hypoxia, infarct, or pericarditis. Depression may indicate myocardial hypoxia, infarct, trauma, digoxin toxicity, or alterations in serum potassium (see Chapter 4, ST segment abnormalities).

The T wave is the first deflection after the QRS complex and should be less than $1/4$ the size of the R wave in height. The T wave may be upright or negative or even biphasic. Tall and tented (sharp) T waves may indicate hyperkalemia, which may be a life-threatening emergency (see Chapter 4, T wave abnormalities). Depression or elevation from baseline may indicate myocardial hypoxia, cardiac hypertrophy, or electrolyte alterations (including hyperkalemia). In emergency situations electrolyte measurement should be done to rule out hyperkalemia first, followed by assessment of oxygenation to rule out hypoxia. If the findings are normal then a cardiac consultation is recommended. Low amplitude or inverted T waves may indicate hypokalemia, hypocalcemia, or ischemia. Alternans of the T wave (variation in height with alternating beats) has been reported with hypocalcemia.

The Q-T interval is measured from the beginning of the Q wave to the end of the T wave and represents ventricular depolarization through ventricular repolarization. Ideally it should be less than half of the previous R-R interval in width. A prolonged Q-T interval is not common in dogs and cats but is important as it can degenerate into a potentially fatal arrhythmia called torsade de pointes (see Chapter 3, Torsade de pointes). This is a ventricular rhythm that is a bit more regular than ventricular fibrillation but with a polarity that rotates around the baseline. It seems as if the complexes alternate between taller and shorter complexes and it has been described as resembling ribbon candy. It may occur in brief periods (~5 s) or it may degenerate into ventricular fibrillation. Prolongation of the QT interval can be hereditary in Dalmatian and English Springer Spaniel dogs or can be caused by numerous drugs, hypokalemia, hypocalcemia, or toxicity in other breeds.

A systematic approach to reading ECGs is recommended. This includes calculation of the heart rate (and verifying this with auscultation of the heart and lungs), checking for and minimizing artifacts, evaluating the rhythm (is there a P wave for every QRS, is the rhythm regular, irregular, or irregularly irregular, etc.) and, when the animal is stable, measuring the complexes. The information gained from evaluation of the ECG must be put into context with the species (e.g., sinus arrhythmia is never normal in a cat), the breed (e.g., prolonged QT syndrome in Dalmatian and English Springer Spaniels), the physical examination (e.g., does the heart rate on the ECG and on auscultation match, are there heart beats without concurrent pulses, etc.), and additional diagnostics (e.g., CBC, biochemistry panel, radiographs, echocardiogram, and so on).

The following sections highlight life-threatening arrhythmias and cardiac conditions most likely to be encountered in small animal practice.

Chapter 2 Bradyarrhythmias

Sinus bradycardia

 Recognition

Sinus bradycardia is a regular sinus rhythm with a slow rate. In dogs (especially athletic dogs or large breed dogs) this may be normal. It is abnormal in cats at a veterinary facility (unless well acclimated to the practice) and the presence of a serious underlying disorder (e.g., sepsis, hyperkalemia) should be investigated in cats.

 Differentials and diagnostics

For dogs rule out vagal causes (GI disturbances, respiratory disease), head trauma (Cushing reflex will most likely have hypertension associated with the bradycardia), hypothermia, hypothyroidism, and electrolyte changes (especially hyperkalemia). Drug toxicities can cause this as well (opioids, calcium channel blockers, beta blockers, digoxin, and many others). Most cases in dogs do not warrant treatment if the rate is only slightly below the normal range for that breed. Always address any underlying abnormalities. For cats rule out sepsis (causes bradycardia in cats along with hypotension) and hyperkalemia.

 Treatment

Address underlying cause.

 Prognosis

Excellent if physiologic cause. All else depends on underlying problem.

Life-Threatening Cardiac Emergencies for the Small Animal Practitioner, First Edition. Maureen McMichael and Ryan Fries.
© 2016 John Wiley & Sons, Inc. Published 2016 by John Wiley & Sons, Inc.

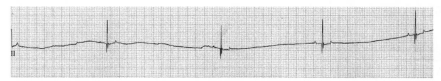

Figure 5 Sinus bradycardia.

Sinus arrhythmia

 Recognition

Alternating periods of faster and then slower heart rates with normal P-QRS complexes. A wandering pacemaker (different amplitudes of the P wave) is often present. Normal in dogs and common in brachycephalic breeds; always abnormal in cats. During a respiratory sinus arrhythmia, the heart rate (HR) increases during inspiration and decreases during expiration due to alterations in vagal tone (+/− low sympathetic tone).

 Differentials and diagnostics

Rule out high vagal tone from GI disease or respiratory disease.

 Treatment

None required for dogs. For cats a full workup to rule out underlying disease is indicated.

 Prognosis

Excellent for normal dogs. Guarded for cats depending on underlying cause.

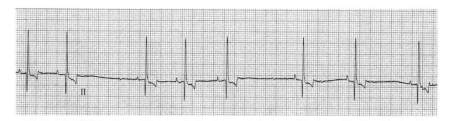

Figure 6 Sinus arrhythmia.

Sinus arrest

 Recognition

A flat line of variable duration in an ECG usually followed by an escape beat. It is due to failure of the SA node to discharge causing a pause (flat line) that is ≥ two times the underlying R-R interval.

 Differentials and diagnostics

Most commonly caused by disorder of the SA node and often associated with bradycardia-tachycardia syndrome (previously called sick sinus syndrome). Can also be caused by drug toxicities or neoplasia.

 Treatment

Address any underlying issues (drug toxicities), reverse any anesthetics. A full cardiac workup is indicated and a pacemaker is usually the only effective treatment in symptomatic patients.

 Prognosis

Depends on underlying cause. Good for dogs treated with pacemaker implantation.

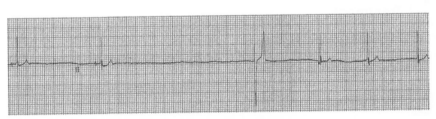

Figure 7 Sinus arrest. Note escape beat following 2nd complex.

Atrial standstill

 Recognition

Absence of P waves, slow HR, can have normal-looking QRS (upright and narrow). If due to hyperkalemia (a common cause) see small to no P wave, slow ventricular rate, tall and tented (wide) T waves, and eventual sinoventricular rhythm with HR 20–40 bpm in dogs (60–100 bpm in cats). It is important to listen to the animal as the T wave may be the same height as the R wave and the ECG may double count.

Differentials and diagnostics

Hyperkalemia and atrial muscular dystrophy/fibrosis (English Springer Spaniel) are common rule outs. Minimum data base (PCV, TS, azo, BG) along with electrolytes should be done first (after ECG). Hyperkalemia can be from urinary obstruction or urinary bladder rupture, acute renal failure, hypoadrenocorticism, or diabetic ketoacidosis crisis.

 Treatment

Treat underlying cause while addressing the arrhythmia. Hyperkalemia is most often associated with urinary abnormalities in small animal patients. Male cats should always be evaluated for urethral obstruction (e.g., firm urinary bladder) or uroabdomen (e.g., the urinary bladder has ruptured) and male dogs should be evaluated for uroabdomen (e.g., from ruptured urinary bladder). Additional causes include trauma, acute renal failure, endocrine disorders (e.g., hypoadrenocorticism, diabetic ketoacidosis), and ruptured ureters. If hyperkalemia is diagnosed or strongly suspected consider treating with calcium gluconate 10% IV at 0.5–1.0 mL/kg over 20 min (not to exceed 10 mL in any animal) while monitoring the ECG. A pacemaker is required for dogs with atrial muscular dystrophy or fibrosis.

 Prognosis

Guarded depending on underlying cause. Guarded to good for dogs with pacemaker implantation.

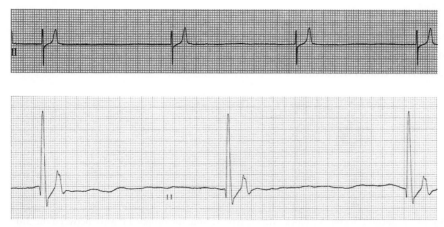

Figures 8 and 9 Atrial standstill.

AV BLOCK OVERVIEW

First-degree AV block

 Recognition

Prolonged P-R interval. Often vagal induced. Usually treatment of primary cause is all that is needed.

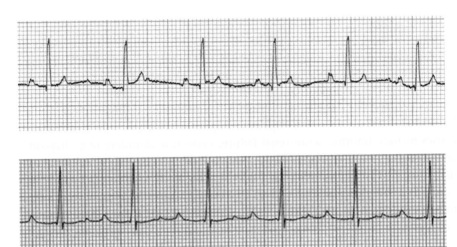

Figures 10 and 11 First-degree AV block.

Second-degree AV block

Mobitz type 1 (Wenckebach)

 Recognition

P-R interval prolongs until a block occurs (P wave without a QRS following it). As in first-degree block rule out high vagal tone and usually treatment of underlying cause is all that is needed.

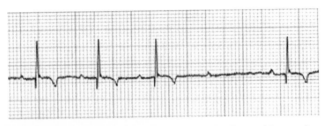

Figure 12 Second-degree AV block, Mobitz type 1. Note the dropped P wave between the 3rd and 4th complexes.

Mobitz type 2

 Recognition

Blocked P waves (P waves without QRS following it, there are more P waves than QRS complexes) with normal or abnormal morphology of QRS complexes. P-R interval is consistent (but may be prolonged). Usually the result of primary cardiac conduction abnormality or drug toxicity. Degree of block can be highly variable and it can progress to third degree.

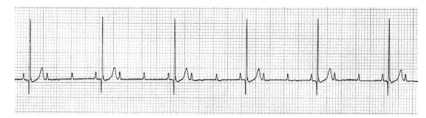

Figure 13 Second-degree AV block, Mobitz type 2.

Third-degree AV block

 Recognition

P waves are independent of (e.g., dissociated from) QRS complexes and there is a slow ventricular rate. QRS morphology may appear normal if the escape pacemaker is above the bundle of His and there is no bundle branch block. There is an abnormal morphology to the QRS complexes (e.g., they are wide and bizarre) if the escape pacemaker is below the AV junction with bundle branch block or of ventricular origin. This is usually the result of a primary cardiac conduction disturbance.

 Differentials and diagnostics

A minimum data base (PCV, TS, azo, BG), CBC, biochemistry panel, blood gas, CXR, echocardiogram.

Rule out non-cardiac causes including hyperkalemia, excess vagal tone (e.g., from respiratory disease, brachycephalic syndrome, GI disease), hypothyroidism, decompensated shock or sepsis (especially cats), increased intracranial pressure, hypothermia, acid-base abnormalities, and drug toxicities. Maybe also consider Chagas titers, tick titers, and cardiac troponin I.

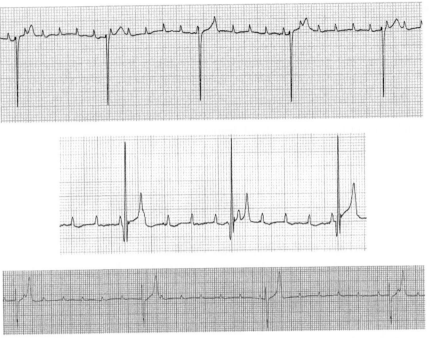

Figures 14–16 Third-degree AV block. All traces show complete AV dissociation. The escape rate and morphology can vary depending on the origin of the escape (junction = narrow QRS, ventricle = wide QRS).

 Treatment

Must treat any underlying cause.

Pacemaker

Treatment of choice for second-degree AV block type 2 and third-degree AV block is a pacemaker.

Atropine

Do not use atropine when the animal is significantly hypothermic (re-warming will increase HR), in shock, or in a hypothyroid crisis. In other cases, if life-threatening bradycardia is affecting perfusion, give atropine 0.04 mg/kg IV.

Repeat ECG in 3–5 min.

If no response consider glycopyrrolate (0.005–0.01 mg/kg IV).

If no response consider isoproterenol (0.04 μg/kg/min as CRI; side effects include: ventricular arrhythmias, hypotension, vomiting, and tachycardia).

If isoproterenol fails try dopamine (4–6 μg/kg/min up to 7–15 μg/kg/min).

Hyperkalemia

If bradycardia is secondary to hyperkalemia give 10% calcium gluconate (0.5 to 1.0 mL/kg slow IV while watching ECG; up to a max of 10 mL in any animal) for cardioprotection.

Specific therapy for hyperkalemia is to treat the underlying cause (e.g., urethral obstruction, uroabdomen, acute renal failure, hypoadrenocorticism, etc.). After calcium gluconate can give 50% dextrose at 0.5–1 mL/kg IV diluted 1:4 with 0.9% NaCl to increase insulin to carry potassium intracellularly. See emergency texts for additional treatments (e.g., insulin, sodium bicarbonate).

 Prognosis

Depends on degree of heart block—good for first-degree and second-degree type 1, variable to poor without pacemaker implantation for second-degree type 2 and third degree as these atrioventricular conduction defects have been associated with syncope and sudden death.

Asystole

 Recognition

Complete absence of depolarization and contraction, showing a flat line on the ECG. This is a terminal rhythm and needs to be addressed with CPR immediately (see CPR).

 Differentials and diagnostics

Always verify the ECG (check leads, machine, etc.) and the patient (listen to the heart, palpate pulses) as occasionally a flat line is due to faulty (or disconnected equipment).

 Treatment

CPR if no heart beat on auscultation.

 Prognosis

Poor to guarded depending on underlying cause.

Cardiopulmonary arrest

The RECOVER (Reassessment Campaign on Veterinary Resuscitation initiative) guidelines for veterinary CPR are available free at www.veccs.org. The guidelines stress the importance of decreasing interruption of chest compressions and avoiding hyperventilation.

I. Airway: Establish airway via endotracheal tube or emergency tracheostomy.

II. Breathing: Ventilate with 100% oxygen at 10 bpm using tidal volume of 10 mL/kg (ventilator) or peak airway pressure of 20 cmH_2O. Do not over ventilate.

III. Circulation: First establish arrest, check for pulses, heart sounds, and if absent proceed. Begin compressions in lateral recumbency at a rate of 100–120 compressions per min. Chest compression depth of 1/3 to 1/2 the width of the chest is the goal, allow full chest recoil between compressions. Simultaneously have another person place a large gauge over-the-needle IV catheter (percutaneous or via cut-down) in a central vein (jugular or saphenous) or in a peripheral vein if unable to place in central vein. Collect blood from hub of catheter for HCT, TS, azo, BG, if possible check electrolytes, lactate and venous blood gas and correct any specific abnormalities (e.g., hypoglycemia, hypokalemia, and so on).

IV. Monitor perfusion with end tidal CO_2 (as CO_2 increases perfusion is improving). A higher $ETCO_2$ correlates with improved survival in humans. Consider open chest CPR early (see below).

V. Drugs: **Epinephrine @ 0.01 mg/kg IV first dose** (low dose; double dose if through endotracheal route and dilute 1:1 with 0.9% NaCl; administer via catheter longer than the endotracheal tube). Repeat in 3–5 min and if no response after prolonged arrest, give epinephrine at 0.1 mg/kg IV (high dose) for subsequent doses (double if through trachea and dilute 1:1 with 0.9% NaCl). Consider **arginine vasopressin @ 0.8 U/kg (0.2 mL per 10 pounds of 20 U/mL concentration)** as a substitute or in combination with epinephrine q3–5min. See specific arrhythmias below for additional drug dosages. Alkalinization with sodium bicarbonate at 1 mEq/kg after prolonged arrest >10–15 min may be considered but is controversial.

VI. Reversal agents: If reversible anesthetic/sedative medication has been given, administer reversal agent during CPR. For α-2 agonists (dexmedetomidine, xylazine), consider atipamezole (0.2 mg/kg IM, IV) or yohimbine (0.1 mg/kg IV dogs), respectively; for benzodiazepines (diazepam, midazolam), consider flumazenil (0.01 mg/kg IV); for full mu opioids (hydromorphone, morphine, fentanyl, etc.) consider naloxone (0.01–0.02 mg/kg IM, IV).

VII. **ECG rhythm**:
   a. **Asystole**: Recognized as absence of any complexes on ECG or "flat line." Treat with atropine @ 0.04 mg/kg IV if associated with high vagal tone or excessive vagal stimulation or epinephrine @ 0.01 mg/kg IV first dose and q3–5min if there is no association with high vagal tone. In dogs and cats, routine use of atropine during arrest may be considered along with epinephrine. Use for asystole, also pulseless electrical activity (PEA).
   b. **Ventricular tachycardia (VT)**: Usually seen post resuscitation and can be treated with lidocaine bolus @ 2–4 mg/kg IV in dogs and 0.2 mg/kg in cats. If successful a lidocaine CRI @ 25–75 μg/kg/min in dogs and 10–40 μg/kg/min in cats can be started. **Caution lidocaine toxicity in cats!** Procainamide (1–2 mg/kg slow IV) preferred for cats.
   c. **Ventricular fibrillation (VF)**: Can be either fine (lower amplitude) or coarse (higher amplitude with more orderly appearance). Coarse VF may be easier to convert to sinus rhythm than fine VF. VF is more responsive early and should be identified as early as possible. Epinephrine can improve the responsiveness of VF to defibrillation. The treatment is electrical defibrillation at a dose of 4–6 joules/kg (using a monophasic defibrillator) and 2–4 joules/kg (using a biphasic defibrillator) for external defibrillation. One-tenth the calculated dose can be used for internal defibrillation. Conduction paste is used on paddles (**NEVER ALCOHOL**), with the patient in dorsal recumbency. Paddles are placed on opposite side of the chest, pressure is applied, and when defibrillator is charged "CLEAR" is called. No one can be in contact with the animal or the table during defibrillation or they will get shocked, this includes the resuscitator and the hanging stethoscope around their neck. After defibrillation compressions are immediately resumed for 2 min before checking the rhythm. If VF persists another shock is delivered (the dose should be increased once by 50–100% for refractory VF/pulseless VT) and compressions are resumed for 2 min before checking rhythm. If VF still persists consider magnesium sulfate @ 30 mg/kg (0.2–0.3 mEq/kg) slow IV (over 20 min). Chemical defibrillation consists of 1 mmol/kg KCl IV followed by epinephrine @ 0.1 mg/kg IV and is rarely successful.
   d. **Electromechanical dissociation**: Defined as a normal-looking to bizarre ECG rhythm with no mechanical activity (i.e., the heart is not beating, there are no heart sounds and no pulses). Treatment consists of epinephrine @ 0.01 mg/kg IV for the first dose often in combination with atropine at 0.04 mg/kg IV if high vagal tone or can consider vasopressin.

VIII. **Fluids**: For euvolemic or hypervolemic dogs and cats, the routine administration of IV fluids is not recommended. If the animal was hypovolemic prior to arrest, an isotonic crystalloid bolus can be administered at:

Dogs: 20 mL/kg (up to 90 mL/kg), Cats: 10 mL/kg (up to 45 mL/kg) followed by reassessment of perfusion (urine output, lactate, extremity temperature, pulse quality, mentation).

If minimal improvement, consider synthetic colloids (HES):

Dogs: 5 mL/kg bolus over 15–20 min and reassess perfusion. Give up to 20 mL/kg total.

Cats: 2–5 mL/kg bolus over 20–30 min and reassess perfusion. Colloids should not be bolused rapidly to cats. Give up to 10 mL/kg in total.

Red blood cells and plasma are given if indicated.

IX. **Open chest CPR**: Indicated in large dogs and animals with pneumothorax, chest trauma, pleural effusion, pericardial effusion, diaphragmatic hernia, dogs currently undergoing surgery or in cases where there is no evidence of circulation (pulses) after 5 min of starting compressions and the owner has consented to this.

Procedure:

A quick clip of one strip of hair at left 5–6th intercostal space is done followed by a quick swab once with non-alcohol antiseptic. An incision midway between ribs down to pleura is made while avoiding the internal thoracic artery (runs 1 cm lateral to sternum), and rib vessels. This is followed by blunt penetration into pleura with curved mayo scissors (between ventilations), and extending the incision dorsally and ventrally. The pericardium is opened (avoid the phrenic nerve which lies over the heart), and the heart is compressed from apex to base at rate of 100–120 bpm. Small hearts can be compressed with one hand, larger hearts need both hands (do not rotate heart and kink vessels). As compressions begin, filling of the ventricle should be felt, followed by another compression. If ventricular filling is not appreciated consider more volume (i.e., IV fluids). If CPR is successful, part of the pericardium is removed (careful not to incise phrenic nerve) because pericardial effusion is common post open chest CPR. This is followed by warm sterile chest lavage, chest tube placement, closing of the incision, and antibiotic administration. Analgesia is started as soon as possible when the animal begins to awaken.

X. **Post resuscitation care**: Frequent or continuous monitoring of pulse oximetry, arterial blood gas ($PaCO_2$ as indicator of ventilation) and acid-base status, electrolytes, continuous ECG, blood pressure (preferably direct), Hct, TS, BG, azo, body temperature, urine output, CVP and lactate are essential. The following should be avoided: hyperglycemia, hyperthermia, and hypoventilation. Ventilation is done manually or via

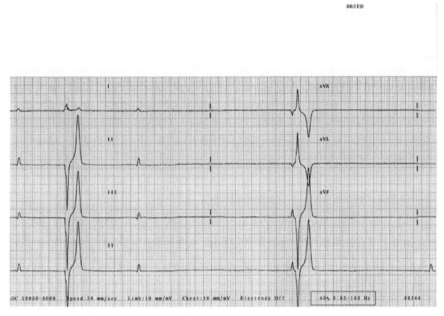

Figure 17 Pulseless electrical activity.

machine until appropriate spontaneous ventilations return. The $PaCO_2$ is maintained between 32–43 mmHg dogs and 26–36 mmHg cats and PaO_2 >80 mmHg. Systolic blood pressure should be >90 mmHg and supplemental oxygen should be continued after spontaneous ventilations return. Common post CPR abnormalities include reperfusion injury, cerebral edema, cardiac arrhythmias, hypoxemia, acute renal failure. Correct underlying cause of CPR.

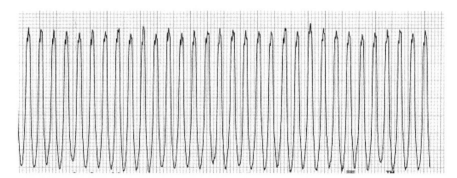

Figure 18 Pulseless ventricular tachycardia.

Escape rhythms

 Recognition

Rate is slower than SA node rate (normal HR) for that species but this may be deceptive on ECG which can occasionally duplicate the rate (machine reads tallest wave as R wave, if T wave is tall it can double count). Always verify the rate with auscultation. If junctional escape beats, the QRS will be upright and narrow. If ventricular escape beats, the QRS is wide and bizarre and the rate can be very slow (20–40 bpm).

 Differentials and diagnostics

A minimum data base (PCV, TS, azo, BG) with electrolytes (always check potassium) and ECG should be done first. Major rule outs here are hyperkalemia

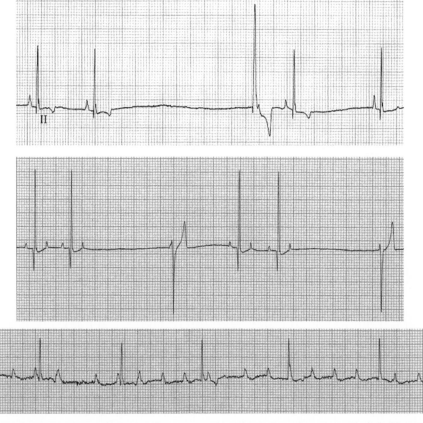

Figures 19–21 Escape rhythm. Note the escape beats in the first two traces after the pause in sinus rhythm. The bottom trace shows complete AV dissociation and a narrow, relatively fast escapse rhythm (junctional escape).

and third-degree AV block. See Electrolyte section for specifics on diagnosing and treating hyperkalemia. See AV block for specifics on diagnosing and treating third-degree AV block. Escape rhythms occur when the pacemaker with the highest rate (SA node) stops working or only works intermittently. Escape rhythms should be thought of as rescue rhythms—they are protective and should never be suppressed. This is an attempt by the pacemaker cells downstream to initiate a rhythm when the pacemaker upstream stops working. General order is SA node, AV node/junction, ventricle (Purkinje fibers). If SA fails, AV node/junction should initiate an escape rhythm and if the AV fails the ventricle should initiate one. Each successive move down the chain is associated with a slower HR, with AV junctional rates of 40–60 bpm in the dog and ventricular rates of 20–40 bpm in the dog. Cat rates are much higher and can be deceptive and easily missed as an escape rhythm. In the cat AV junctional rates can be as high as 140 bpm and ventricular rates as high as 80 bpm.

 Treatment

Always treat the underlying problem, do not suppress this protective rhythm. If hyperkalemia present consider calcium gluconate 10% at 0.5–1.0 mL/kg IV over 20 min while monitoring the ECG (to a max of 10 mL in any animal) and while addressing the underlying issue (uroabdomen, urethral obstruction, and so on). If third-degree AV block consider immediate referral to cardiologist for workup and pacemaker.

 Prognosis

Good if underlying issue addressed or if pacemaker can be implanted.

Chapter 3 Tachyarrhythmias

Atrial premature complexes

 Recognition

Atrial premature complexes (APC) are easy to miss as they have normal QRS morphology (upright, narrow) and are just early (premature). The average HR is often normal, but the rhythm is irregular due to the APC. The APC P wave may be negative, positive, biphasic, or may be superimposed on the T wave preceding it.

 Differentials and diagnostics

May be indicative of cardiac abnormality in dogs and cats or less frequently systemic disease. Cardiac workup to include baseline CBC, biochemistry panel, ECG, CXR, and echocardiogram is recommended.

 Treatment

Treat the underlying heart disease.

 Prognosis

Depends on underlying heart disease.

Life-Threatening Cardiac Emergencies for the Small Animal Practitioner, First Edition. Maureen McMichael and Ryan Fries.
© 2016 John Wiley & Sons, Inc. Published 2016 by John Wiley & Sons, Inc.

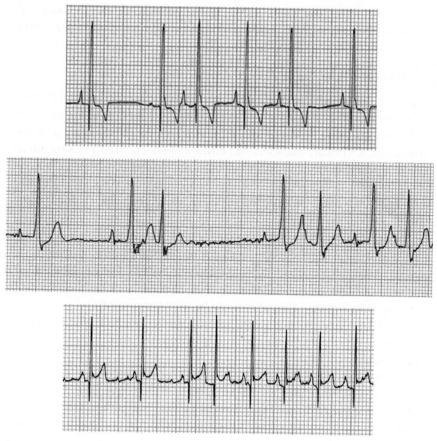

Figures 22, 23 and 24 Atrial premature complexes. In the first tracing the 3rd complex is an APC, in the second tracing the 3rd, 5th, and 7th complexes are APCs, and in the last tracing the 4th complex is an APC.

Ventricular premature complexes

 Recognition

Wide and bizarre QRS complexes with no association with the P wave preceding it. Often followed by a pause.

 Differentials and diagnostics

Ventricular premature complexes (VPC) are indicative of disease or ischemia in a portion of the ventricle and may, if frequent enough, lead to poor perfusion. In dogs these often occur due to non-cardiac causes such as GDV, splenic disease, sepsis, and trauma. Also seen commonly in large breed dogs with underlying cardiac disease and in Boxers with ARVC. Minimum database (PCV, TS, azo, BG), CBC, biochemistry panel, ECG, CXR, and echocardiogram should be performed.

 ## Treatment in dogs

In dogs with non-cardiac disease treat the underlying disorder, paying particular attention to acid-base and electrolyte abnormalities, perfusion optimization, and adequate analgesia. In dogs with cardiac disease treat the underlying cardiac abnormalities. If VPCs are not affecting perfusion do not treat. If VPCs are affecting perfusion, or are frequent with R on T morphology treat with the following:
- Lidocaine bolus (2–4 mg/kg IV) if sustained VT at rate >180 bpm and affecting perfusion (urine output, lactate, extremity temperature, pulse quality, mentation).
  - If successful follow with lidocaine CRI (25–75 µg/kg/min).
  - Keep potassium normalized; lidocaine is not effective if hypokalemic.
- Consider magnesium sulfate (1.0–2.0 mEq/kg/day IV CRI or magnesium sulfate bolus at 30 mg/kg [0.3 mEq/kg] over 20 min IV). Reduce dose by 50% if azotemic. Lidocaine and magnesium can be used concurrently.
- Nausea or vomiting may indicate lidocaine toxicity. Stop lidocaine and verify the dosage. If correct, decrease the dose by $\frac{1}{2}$ and start again.
- Procainamide
  If lidocaine is unsuccessful try procainamide (5–15 mg/kg over 10 min IV). Follow with procainamide CRI (25–50 µg/kg/min).
- With refractory arrhythmias consider lidocaine and procainamide.
- *Or* esmolol (0.5 mg/kg slow IV) follow with an esmolol CRI (50–200 µg/kg/min).
- *Or* propranolol (0.02–0.06 mg/kg slow IV or IM q8h), beta blockers can significantly decrease cardiac output and should be used with extreme caution.

 ## Treatment in cats

Do not start anti-arrhythmics unless HR >240 bpm (by auscultation, not just on ECG) and affecting perfusion.

Due to lidocaine toxicity in cats start with procainamide (3–8 mg/kg over 10 min IV 1-2 mg/kg IV) or propranolol (0.25–0.5 mg/per cat over 10 min IV or IM). If lidocaine is necessary, use 0.25–1.0 mg/kg followed by a CRI @ 10–40 µg/kg/min.

Watch for seizures.

 ## Prognosis

Good for non-cardiac causes if the underlying disorder is addressed. Poor to guarded for primary cardiac disease.

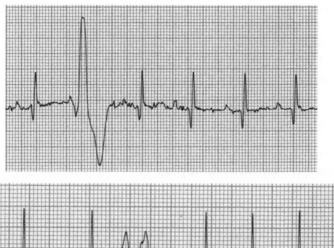

Figures 25 and 26 Ventricular premature complexes.

Differentiating SVT from VT

With supraventricular tachycardia (SVT) the QRS complexes are upright and typ-ically narrow and the rate is rapid. With typical ventricular tachycardia (VT) the QRS complexes are wide and bizarre as the initiation of the impulse is coming from below the AV node. However, there are arrhythmias that are supraventric-ular in origin but resemble VT. These are called SVT with aberrancy and can be very difficult (even for cardiologists) to differentiate. In humans they are called wide complex tachycardia (WCT). These arise when an SVT occurs in an animal with a conduction abnormality such as bundle branch block. There are several ways to attempt to distinguish between the two arrhythmias.

More likely VT if,

- Capture beats are present
  These occur when the SA node transiently captures the beat to produce a QRS of normal duration. It resembles a normal-looking QRS among a sea of wide, bizarre complexes.
- Fusion beats are present

These occur when the sinus beat and the ventricular beat occur simultaneously to produce a hybrid complex.
- AV dissociation is present
  The P and QRS complexes occur at different rates.
- Lidocaine (dogs) or procainamide (cats) terminates the rhythm.

More likely SVT with aberration if,

- P waves have a consistent relationship to QRS
- Vagal maneuver terminates the rhythm

 ## Treatment in general

When a WCT cannot be distinguished as either VT or SVT with aberrancy, it is best to treat for VT. There are several reasons for this; VT is much more common than SVT with aberrancy, lidocaine (in dogs) or procainamide are safer options if it is not VT, and drugs used to treat SVT (calcium channel blockers) can cause hypotension, which can be detrimental if the animal is in VT.

 ## Treatment in dogs

Lidocaine bolus (2–4 mg/kg IV) if sustained VT at rate >180 bpm and affecting perfusion (urine output, lactate, extremity temperature, pulse quality, mentation).
- If successful follow with lidocaine CRI (25–75 µg/kg/min).
- Keep potassium normalized; lidocaine is not effective if hypokalemic.
- Consider magnesium sulfate (1.0–2.0 mEq/kg/day IV CRI or magnesium sulfate bolus at 30 mg/kg [0.3 mEq/kg] over 20 min IV). Reduce dose by 50% if azotemic. Lidocaine and magnesium can be used concurrently.
- Nausea or vomiting may indicate lidocaine toxicity. Stop lidocaine and verify the dosage. If correct, decrease the dose by $\frac{1}{2}$ and start again.
- Procainamide
  If lidocaine unsuccessful try procainamide (5–15 mg/kg over 10 min IV). Follow with procainamide CRI (25–50 µg/kg/min).
- With refractory arrhythmias consider lidocaine and procainamide.
- *Or* esmolol (0.5 mg/kg slow IV) follow with an esmolol CRI (50–200 µg/kg/min).
- *Or* propranolol (0.02–0.06 mg/kg slow IV or IM q8h), beta blockers can significantly decrease cardiac output and should be used with extreme caution.

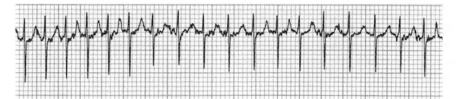

Figure 27 Supraventricular Tachycardia.

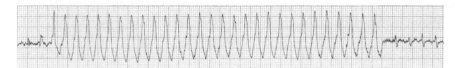

Figure 28 Ventricular Tachycardia.

 ## Treatment in cats

Do not start anti-arrhythmics unless HR >240 bpm (by auscultation, not just on ECG) and affecting perfusion.

Due to lidocaine toxicity in cats start with procainamide (3–8 mg/kg over 10 min IV 1-2 mg/kg IV) or propranolol (0.25–0.5 mg/per cat over 10 min IV or IM). If lidocaine is necessary, use 0.25–1.0 mg/kg followed by a CRI @ 10–40 µg/kg/min.

Watch for seizures.

 ## Prognosis

Good for non-cardiac causes if the underlying disorder is addressed. Poor to guarded for primary cardiac disease.

Supraventricular tachycardia

 ## Recognition

Rapid HR with upright, narrow QRS complexes. SVT refers to a rapid rhythm that originates above the bundle of HIS. This section will cover all SVT except atrial fibrillation, which will be covered in the next section. Rhythm may be more regular than that of atrial fibrillation.

 ## Differentials and diagnostics

Dog or cat may be clinically normal or show varying degrees of weakness, collapse, pale to cyanotic mucous membranes, pulse deficits, irregular "chaotic"

rhythm or respiratory abnormalities. Identify P waves, if none seen do a six-lead ECG, if wide and bizarre QRS complexes consider VT. Look for other clues for VT (e.g., fusion beats, AV dissociation). Once supraventricular tachycardia is confirmed then differentiate between atrial tachycardia and sinus tachycardia. Can try vagal maneuver (firm pressure on eyeballs or deep carotid massage) to slow the heart rate. An abrupt termination of the tachycardia suggests atrial tachycardia, while a gradual slowing down of the rate suggests sinus tachycardia. Vagal maneuvers are often unsuccessful. If the SVT has an irregularly irregular rhythm it is likely to be atrial fibrillation (see "Atrial fibrillation" section later).

- Minimum data base (PCV, TS, azo, BG), CBC, biochemistry panel, CXR, and echocardiogram should be done when stable. Rule out drug toxicity (i.e., digoxin) and causes of sinus tachycardia (e.g., pain, anxiety, hyperthermia, hyperthyroidism, hypovolemia, hypoxia, electrolyte abnormalities).

 ## Treatment

- Oxygen supplementation
- IV catheter
- Diltiazem
  If HR >180 bpm and affecting perfusion (urine output, lactate, extremity temperature, pulse quality, mentation), give diltiazem (0.25 mg/kg over 10 min IV) to slow ventricular response to atrial tachycardia (including atrial fibrillation and flutter) over 10 minutes, through a peripheral vein.
  - Follow with diltiazem CRI (1–5 µg/kg/min).
- *Or* procainamide (10–15 mg/kg IV over 5–10 min, to effect, followed by a CRI @ 25–50 µg/kg/min).
- Diltiazem has negative inotropic effects (can decrease cardiac output); perfusion must be carefully monitored. Procainamide can cause vasodilation and hypotension when given rapidly.
- If congestive heart present failure, give furosemide (2 mg/kg IV).
- If cardiogenic shock (very decreased urine output, cold extremities, increased lactate) dobutamine is administered (2.5 µg/kg/min) increasing the infusion every 30 min until systolic pressure is >90 mmHg. Typical end point is 5–10 µg/kg/min. Once BP is stable (systolic BP > 90 mmHg), consider applying nitroglycerin paste ($\frac{1}{2}$ inch to shaved portion of thorax or ear pinnae) or sodium nitroprusside @ 0.5–3 µg/kg/min IV CRI. Start at lowest dose of nitroprusside and titrate up q15–30min depending on clinical response. Monitor blood pressure as severe hypotension can result. Stop nitroprusside when MAP < 60 mmHg or systolic blood pressure is <90 mmHg. Drug is light-sensitive—cover line and bag. Cyanide toxicity if overdose or rapid bolus—label line and catheter "DO NOT FLUSH."
- Young Labradors with congenital SVT: catheter ablation may be treatment of choice.

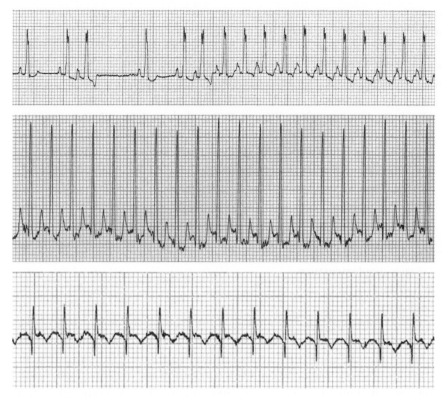

Figures 29, 30 and 31 Supraventricular tachycardia.

 Prognosis

Depends on underlying cause.

Atrial fibrillation

 Recognition

Lack of identifiable P waves, rapid rate, and an irregularly, irregular rhythm (use calipers).

 Differentials and diagnostics

Usually giant/large breed dogs, may have concurrent dilated cardiomyopathy (DCM). Often acute onset lethargy, weakness, exercise intolerance. In cats usually associated with severe underlying cardiomyopathy. Owner may mention something is wrong with the heart, as they may be able to palpate the arrhythmia. May have any or all of the following: weakness, abdominal fluid wave (ascites), pale to cyanotic mucous membranes, tachycardia with chaotic heart sounds (very irregular), weak pulses, pulse deficits, and hypothermia. Often pulse rate much lower than heart rate. Clinical signs depend on ventricular rate. There is loss of atrial kick (atrial contraction) so cardiac output is decreased.

- Minimum data base (PCV, TS, azo, BG) and electrolytes, ECG (tachycardia with irregularly irregular rhythm, no visible P waves, usually upright, narrow QRS). Also consider lactate, CXR (cardiomegaly, pleural effusion, pulmonary edema), echocardiogram (underlying heart disease), CBC, biochemistry panel, UA, thyroid panel, taurine level.

 Treatment in dogs

- Oxygen supplementation
- IV catheter
- Diltiazem
  To slow ventricular rate if HR > 180 bpm and affecting perfusion @ 0.25 mg/kg IV over 10 min through a peripheral vein, followed by a CRI @ 1–5 µg/kg/min. Caution must be used when giving this drug to a patient in heart failure or cardiogenic shock. Diltiazem can worsen perfusion and dramatically slow HR, therefore it should be given slowly and only to effect. Stop the infusion if bradycardia or hypotension is observed.
- *Or* procainamide (10–15 mg/kg IV over 5–10 min, to effect), follow with a CRI @ 25–50 µg/kg/min.
- Oral medication
  In less emergent cases try oral medications and start oral medications in all when stable:
  - Diltiazem XR (2–4 mg/kg orally q12h); non sustained-release formulation: diltiazem (0.5–1 mg/kg orally q8h).
- *Or* digoxin (0.005–0.01 mg/kg orally q12h) and check levels in 5–7 days.
- If no response combine diltiazem with digoxin.
- If no response add beta blocker or consider amiodarone:
  - Propranolol (0.2–1 mg/kg orally q8h).
  - *Or* sotalol (1–2 mg/kg orally q12h).
  - *Or* amiodarone (10–20 mg/kg orally q24h for 7 days, then reduced to 3–15 mg/kg orally q24–48h chronically).
- Monitor perfusion (urine output, extremity temp, lactate) while using any of the above drugs (they can decrease cardiac output).
- Congestive heart failure
  If concurrent CHF give furosemide (2 mg/kg IV) and consider nitroglycerin paste $\frac{1}{2}$ inch applied to shaved area of thorax or ear pinnae.
- Cardiogenic shock

If cardiogenic shock (no urine output, cold extremities, increased lactate) dobutamine is administered (2.5 μg/kg/min) increasing the infusion every 30 min until systolic pressure is >90 mmHg. Typical end point is 5–10 μg/kg/min. Once BP is stable (systolic BP > 90 mmHg), consider applying nitroglycerin paste ($\frac{1}{2}$ inch to shaved portion of thorax or ear pinnae) or sodium nitroprusside @ 0.5–3 μg/kg/min IV CRI. Start at lowest dose of nitroprusside and titrate up q15–30min depending on clinical response. Monitor blood pressure as severe hypotension can result. Stop nitroprusside when MAP < 60 mmHg or systolic BP is <90 mmHg. Drug is light-sensitive—cover line and bag. Cyanide toxicity if overdose or rapid bolus—label line and catheter "DO NOT FLUSH."

- Caution with dobutamine!

Can cause tachyarrhythmias which could be fatal; it is essential that diltiazem and/or digoxin be administered first before considering use of dobutamine.

 ## Treatment in cats

- Decrease stress
- Oxygen supplementation
- IV catheter
- Diltiazem (0.25 mg/kg IV over 10 min through a peripheral vein) if HR > 280 bpm and decreased perfusion (urine output, extremity temperature, pulse deficits).
- Congestive heart failure: give furosemide @ 2 mg/kg IV or IM, nitroglycerin paste $\frac{1}{4}$ inch applied to shaved area of thorax or ear pinnae.

 ## Prognosis

Guarded depending on underlying cause.

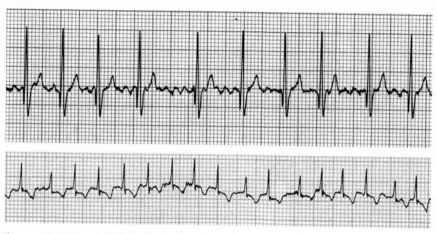

Figures 32, 33, 34 and 35 Atrial fibrillation.

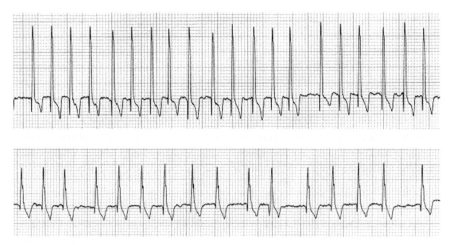

Figures 32, 33, 34 and 35 (*Continued*)

Ventricular pre-excitation

 Recognition

Normal rate and rhythm with upright and wide QRS complexes. Often a delta wave is present which can be identified as a notch on the upstroke of the R wave due to asynchronous activation of the ventricles. Impulses from the atria or SA node activate the ventricle prematurely via an accessory pathway (bypass tract), the rest of the ventricle is activated through the AV node and conduction system.

 Differentials and diagnostics

This occurs when a normal impulse that comes from the SA node splits with part of it going through the AV node and part of it going through a pathway (called an accessory pathway) into the ventricles. This results in the ventricle being "pre-excited" by the part of the impulse that did not go through the AV node. In most cases there are minimal to no clinical signs. A premature atrial depolarization can cause a re-entry (also called Wolff-Parkinson-White syndrome or orthodromic AV reentrant tachycardia (OAVRT); see following section) rhythm and severe tachycardia.

Consider minimum data base (PCV, TS, azo, BG), electrolytes, CXR, echocardiogram, CBC, biochemistry panel.

 Treatment

Treatment is only required if re-entry SVT develops (see below).

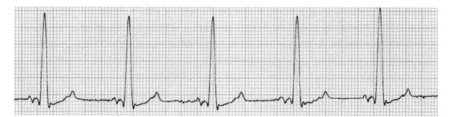

Figure 36 Ventricular pre-excitation. Note the abnormal appearance of the PR interval, delta wave associated with pre-excitation of the ventricle.

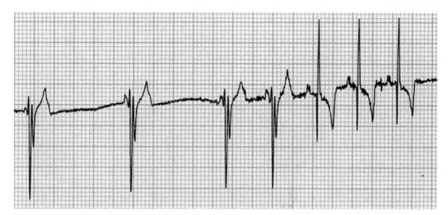

Figure 37 Ventricular pre-excitation. Note the lack of a normal PR interval and aberrant ventricular conduction on the first 4 complexes (pre-excited ventricle).

 Prognosis

Excellent to good if no evidence of SVT or clinical signs. Guarded for dogs with SVT treated medically, good to excellent for dogs treated successfully by catheter ablation.

Re-entrant tachycardia

 Recognition

The HR can be greater than 300 bpm in dogs and is a supraventricular tachycardia. The rhythm is usually regular with upright QRS complexes and a rapid rate. See earlier section "Ventricular pre-excitation" for pathophysiology.

 Differentials and diagnostics

This occurs when a premature atrial depolarization is conducted through the AV node in the normal direction (orthodromic), but is blocked in the accessory pathway. After the ventricle has depolarized the activation may now travel retrograde through the accessory pathway to activate the atria and then conduct through the AV node in the normal direction, setting up an endless loop of conduction. This rhythm is associated with sustained severe tachycardia.

- Consider minimum data base (PCV, TS, azo, BG), electrolytes, CXR, echocardiogram, CBC, biochemistry panel.

 Treatment

Vagal maneuver may break the cycle by slowing AV conduction. Drugs that can be used to treat OAVRT include:

- Diltiazem
  To slow conduction through AV node and break rhythm @ 0.25 mg/kg IV over 10 min through a peripheral vein, followed by a CRI @ 1–5 µg/kg/min.
- Procainamide @ 15 mg/kg IV over 10 min, to effect, follow with a CRI @ 25–50 µg/kg/min.
- Esmolol @ 0.5 mg/kg IV over 1 min
  Definitive treatment is intracardiac catheter radiofrequency ablation of the re-entry pathway.

 Prognosis

Good to excellent with catheter ablation. Guarded with medical management.

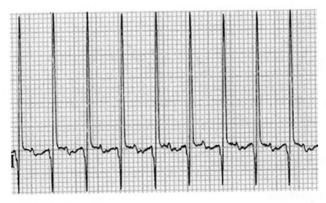

Figure 38 Re-entrant tachycardia.

Wolff-Parkinson-White syndrome

 Recognition

The HR can be greater than 300 bpm in dogs and is a supraventricular tachycardia. The rhythm is usually regular with upright QRS complexes and a rapid rate. See earlier section "Ventricular pre-excitation" for pathophysiology.

Differentials and diagnostics

This occurs when a premature atrial depolarization is conducted through the AV node in the normal direction (orthodromic), but is blocked in the accessory pathway. After the ventricle has depolarized the activation may now travel retrograde through the accessory pathway to activate the atria and then conduct through the AV node in the normal direction, setting up an endless loop of conduction. This rhythm is associated with sustained severe tachycardia.

* Consider minimum data base (PCV, TS, azo, BG), electrolytes, CXR, echocardiogram, CBC, biochemistry panel.

 ## Treatment

Vagal maneuver may break the cycle by slowing AV conduction. Drugs that can be used to treat OAVRT include:
* Diltiazem
  To slow conduction through AV node and break rhythm @ 0.25 mg/kg IV over 10 min through a peripheral vein, followed by a CRI @ 1–5 µg/kg/min.
* Procainamide @ 15 mg/kg IV over 10 min, to effect, follow with a CRI @ 25–50 µg/kg/min.
* Esmolol @ 0.5 mg/kg IV over 1 min.
  Definitive treatment is intracardiac catheter radiofrequency ablation of the re-entry pathway.

 ## Prognosis

Good to excellent with catheter ablation. Guarded with medical management.

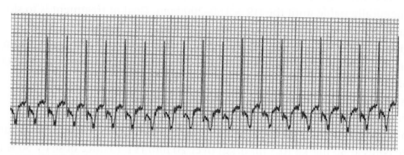

Figure 39 Wolff-Parkinson-White syndrome.

Ventricular tachycardia

 Recognition

Defined as three or more VPCs in a row that are intermittent or sustained and have a rapid rate. History will vary depending on cause. Always rule out non-primary cardiac causes (trauma, shock, sepsis, splenic disease, pancreatitis, neurological disease, GI disease, and hemangiosarcoma). Primary cardiac causes include Boxers with ARVC, Dobermans with underlying cardiac disease, large breed dogs with underlying cardiac disease, and myocarditis. Signs may be related to underlying disease or to primary cardiac disease (e.g. heart murmur, dyspnea, ascites, cachexia). May see pale or cyanotic mucous membranes, prolonged CRT, weak or absent pulses +/- pulse deficits, weakness +/- collapse.

 Differentials and diagnostics

- Minimum data base (PCV, TS, azo, BG), electrolytes (especially ionized magnesium), ECG (tachycardia with wide, bizarre QRS complexes), CBC, biochemistry panel, CXR, arterial or venous blood gas, coagulation panel, echocardiogram. Other diagnostics depend on suspect underlying etiologies (e.g., AUS or abdominal tap for hemoabdomen, right lateral AXR for GDV, and so on). May also consider Chagas titers, tick titers, and cardiac troponin I.

 Treatment in dogs

- Treat any underlying disease.
- Rule out pain (analgesics), hyperthermia, anxiety, anemia or hypovolemia, hypoxia (oxygen supplementation), sepsis, pancreatitis, drug toxicity, electrolyte or acid-base abnormalities. Most dogs with normal hearts will be hemodynamically stable until the HR > 180–200 bpm. Goal of treatment is to slow rate to ~140 bpm or less to maximize perfusion, not eliminate the VT.
- Lidocaine bolus (2–4 mg/kg IV) if sustained VT at rate >180 bpm and affecting perfusion (urine output, lactate, extremity temperature, pulse quality, mentation).
- If successful follow with lidocaine CRI (25–75 µg/kg/min).
- Keep potassium normalized; lidocaine is not effective if hypokalemic.
- Consider magnesium sulfate (1.0–2.0 mEq/kg/day IV CRI or magnesium sulfate bolus at 30 mg/kg [0.3 mEq/kg] over 20 min IV). Reduce dose by 50% if azotemic. Lidocaine and magnesium can be used concurrently.

- Nausea or vomiting may indicate lidocaine toxicity. Stop lidocaine and verify the dosage. If correct, decrease the dose by $\frac{1}{2}$ and start again.
- Procainamide
  If lidocaine unsuccessful try procainamide (5–15 mg/kg over 10 min IV). Follow with procainamide CRI (25–50 µg/kg/min).
- With refractory arrhythmias consider lidocaine and procainamide.
- *Or* esmolol (0.5 mg/kg slow IV) follow with an esmolol CRI (50–200 µg/kg/min).
- *Or* propranolol (0.02–0.06 mg/kg slow IV or IM q8h).
- Beta blockers can significantly decrease cardiac output and should be used with extreme caution.

 ## Treatment in cats

Do not start anti-arrhythmics unless HR > 240 bpm (by auscultation, not just on ECG) and affecting perfusion.

Due to lidocaine toxicity in cats start with procainamide (3–8 mg/kg over 10 min IV 1-2 mg/kg IV) *or* propranolol (0.25–0.5 mg/per cat over 10 min IV or IM). If lidocaine is necessary, use 0.25–1.0 mg/kg followed by a CRI @ 10–40 µg/kg/min.

Watch for seizures.

 ## Prognosis

Depends on underlying cause.

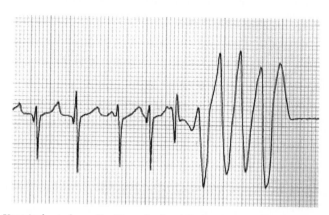

Figure 40 Ventricular tachycardia. Sinus rhythm followed by a paroxsym of R on T ventricular tachycardia.

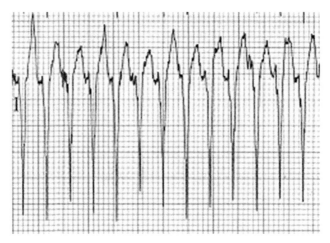

Figure 41 Ventricular tachycardia. Uniform, R on T, ventricular tachycardia.

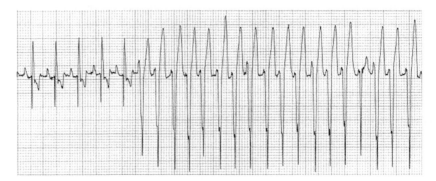

Figure 42 Ventricular tachycardia. Sinus rhythm followed by sustained run of R on T ventricular tachycardia.

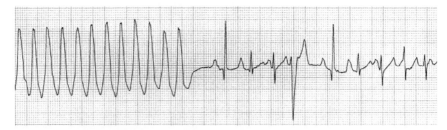

Figure 43 Ventricular tachycardia. Ventricular tachycardia followed by sinus rhythm with frequent fusion complexes.

Accelerated idioventricular rhythm

 Recognition

This is a ventricular rhythm (wide, bizarre complexes) with an intermediate rate. It looks identical to ventricular tachycardia but the rate is slower. Rates generally run between 70–160 bpm in dogs.

 Differentials and diagnostics

Same as for VT (see earlier).

 Treatment

Generally there is less compromise of diastolic filling due to a slower rate. No treatment indicated if perfusion is not compromised. If perfusion is compromised (dull mentation, cold extremities, weak pulses, pale mucous membranes, decreased urine output, etc.) treat as for ventricular tachycardia.

 Prognosis

Guarded.

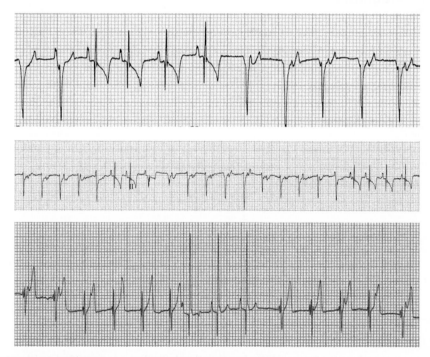

Figures 44, 45 and 46 Accelerated idioventricular rhythm.

Ventricular flutter

 Recognition

This is a rapid ventricular rhythm that may occur before ventricular fibrillation. Alternatively ventricular fibrillation may be recognized without ventricular flutter occurring. It is more organized than ventricular fibrillation but needs to be treated immediately before it degenerates into ventricular fibrillation.

 Differentials and diagnostics

Always distinguish from artifact (check pulses, listen to heart, check ECG leads).

 Treatment

Lidocaine bolus @ 2–4 mg/kg IV in dogs. If successful a lidocaine CRI @ 25–75 µg/kg/min in dogs can be started. **Caution lidocaine toxicity in cats!** Procainamide (1–2 mg/kg slow IV) preferred for cats.

 Prognosis

Poor.

Ventricular fibrillation

 Recognition

This is a rapid, chaotic pattern that does not result in a coordinated contraction of the ventricles. It means the animal has had a cardiopulmonary arrest and CPR must be started immediately.

 Differentials and diagnostics

Distinguish from artifact by checking leads, feeling pulse or listening to heart. Do not delay CPR for this, start CPR immediately.

 Treatment

Start compressions for 2 min while charging the defibrillator. See CPR algorithm.

Prognosis

Poor.

Torsade de pointes

 Recognition

This is a ventricular rhythm that is a bit more regular than ventricular fibrillation but with a polarity that rotates around the baseline. The complexes alternate between taller and shorter and it has been described as resembling ribbon candy. It may occur in brief periods (~5 s) or it may degenerate into ventricular fibrillation.

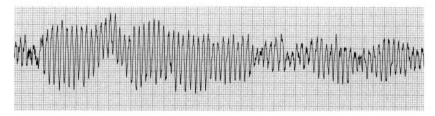

Figure 47 Torsade de pointes.

 Differentials and diagnostics

It is caused by prolongation of the QT interval which can be hereditary in Dalmatian and English Springer Spaniel dogs or can be caused by numerous drugs, hypokalemia, hypocalcemia, or toxicity in other breeds.

 Treatment

Magnesium sulfate @ 30 mg/kg (0.2–0.3 mEq/kg) IV slowly over 20 min. Stop all drugs that may prolong QT interval. Cardiac consult if Dalmatian dog or English Springer Spaniel dog.

 Prognosis

Poor.

Chapter 4 Miscellaneous arrhythmias and cardiac conditions

Artifacts and anomalies

Place all animals in right lateral recumbency for consistency. Always verify lead placement (right forelimb white, left forelimb black, left rear limb red, green is grounding) whenever an arrhythmia is detected. Check machine standardization, which can result in complexes of too large or too small size. Electrical interference (appears as small variations in baseline with high frequency that do not interfere with the QRS complexes) can often be corrected with grounding (attaching the green lead to a grounding element which, by convention, is usually the right hind limb). Artifacts (see Figures 48–50) also occur when the animal moves and are recognized as a changing baseline that is irregular. Other common causes of artifacts include purring, shivering, and electrical interference from cautery machines. Artifacts do not interrupt the normal atrial or ventricular rhythm. Always verify any abnormalities with physical examination.

Arrhythmogenic right ventricular cardiomyopathy

Also called familial ventricular arrhythmia of Boxer dogs, Boxer cardiomyopathy, and arrhythmogenic right ventricular dysplasia. There is no sex predilection and it is suspected to be inherited as an autosomal dominant trait.

 Recognition

Subclinical phase with no clinical signs may occur. During this phase there are no changes on thoracic radiographs or echocardiogram. ECG findings can include typical left bundle branch block-like appearance of VPCs from fibrofatty

Life-Threatening Cardiac Emergencies for the Small Animal Practitioner, First Edition. Maureen McMichael and Ryan Fries.
© 2016 John Wiley & Sons, Inc. Published 2016 by John Wiley & Sons, Inc.

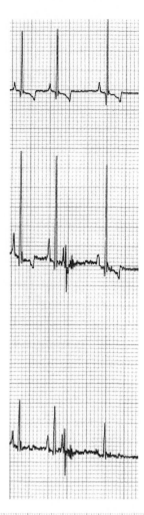

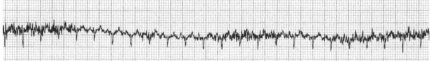

Figures 48–50 Artifact.

replacement of myocytes in the RV. Holter monitor is often needed as some dogs have only 1–2 VPCs per hour. Syncope **or sudden death can occur.**

 Differentials and diagnostics

Routine bloodwork, CXR, echocardiogram, and holter monitor are recommended.

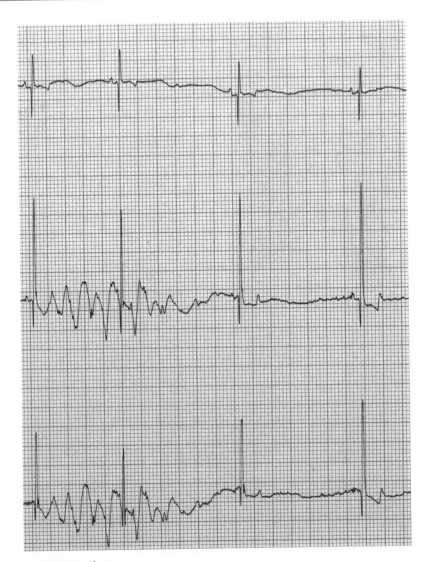

Figures 48–50 Artifact.

 Treatment

Do not breed animals that are diagnosed with ARVC. Treatment is for specific arrhythmias.

 Prognosis

Guarded to good.

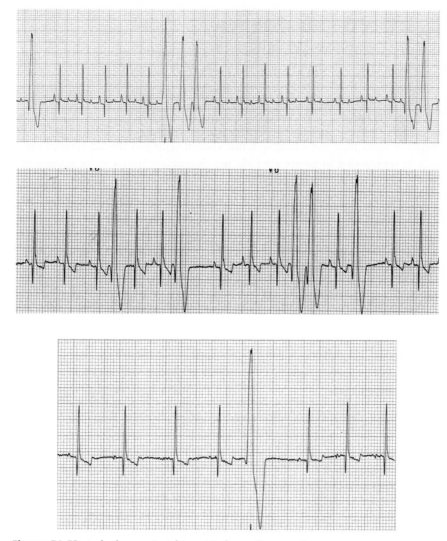

Figures 51–53 Arrhythmogenic right ventricular cardiomyopathy.

AV JUNCTIONAL RHYTHMS

Junctional escape beats

 Recognition

Inverted or absent P wave that occurs before, during or after the QRS. Normal upright QRS, junctional rhythm occurs after a pause in the sinus rhythm and occasionally accelerated or premature.

Differentials and diagnostics

These occur when the AV junctional nodal tissue spontaneously discharges when the SA node fails to discharge creating a pause in normal sinus rhythm.

 Treatment

Junctional beats may not cause systemic clinical signs but should prompt vigilance in monitoring to assure they do not degenerate into a more malignant rhythm. Consider discontinuation or reversal of anesthetics. Do not suppress this rhythm (it is protective). Atropine or glycopyrrolate may re-establish sinus rhythm. Address the underlying condition.

 Prognosis

Guarded.

Junctional rhythm

 Recognition

Inverted or absent P waves, normal upright QRS, slower rate than normal sinus rhythm.

 Differentials and diagnostics

This rhythm occurs when the AV junctional nodal tissue spontaneously discharges during a pause in the sinus rhythm. A continuous junctional rhythm signifies dysfunction of the SA node.

 Treatment

Discontinue or reverse anesthetics, do not suppress this rhythm (it is protective). Atropine or glycopyrrolate may re-establish sinus rhythm. Address the underlying condition.

 Prognosis

Guarded.

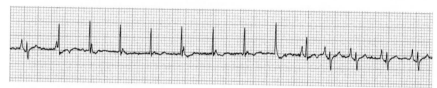

Figure 54 Junctional arrhythmia.

Bradycardia-tachycardia syndrome (sick sinus syndrome)

 Recognition

Miniature Schnauzers, Cocker Spaniels, and West Highland White Terriers predisposed. May have history of syncope. May vary from normal HR, bradycardia, and/or tachycardia. Also called bradycardia-tachycardia syndrome.

 Differentials and diagnostics

ECG (bradycardia, sinoatrial block, may see escape rhythm, paroxysmal tachycardia after bradycardia). A holter monitor is often required to capture the rhythm disturbance as the arrhythmia may be missed during a 3-minute ECG. Additionally a CBC, biochemistry panel, minimum data base (PCV, TS, azo, BG), CXR, and an echocardiogram should be considered.

 Treatment

- Pacemaker is the definitive treatment.
- Atropine
  Life-threatening bradycardia: give atropine (0.04 mg/kg IV) and repeat ECG in 5 min.
  - If no response consider glycopyrrolate (0.005–0.01 mg/kg IV).
  - If no response consider isoproterenol (0.04 µg/kg/min as CRI; side effects include: ventricular arrhythmias, hypotension, vomiting, and tachycardia).
  - If isoproterenol fails try dopamine (4–6 µg/kg/min up to 7–15 µg/kg/min).

 Prognosis

Fair to good with pacemaker.

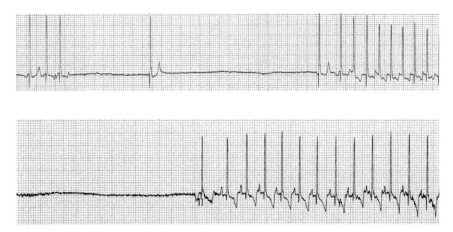

Figures 55 and 56 Bradycardia-tachycardia syndrome (sick sinus syndrome). Note long pauses of sinus arrest.

Electrical alternans (pericardial effusion)

 Recognition

ECG (electrical alternans is a variation in the height of the R wave with every other beat). Small QRS complexes with R wave <1 mV) may also be seen. The history may include weakness, exercise intolerance, collapse, polyuria, polydipsia, vomiting. German Shepherd and Golden Retriever dogs are predisposed. Approximately 19% are idiopathic and 59% are neoplastic. Occasionally other causes are seen such as coagulopathy (anticoagulant rodenticide), ruptured LA, infectious disease, biventricular failure. On physical examination the animal may be weak and have pale to cyanotic mucous membranes, jugular venous distention +/− jugular pulses, muffled heart sounds, weak pulses, pulsus paradoxicus (weaker pulses on inspiration), tachycardia.

 Differentials and diagnostics

ECG, a minimum data base (PCV, TS, azo, BG), CBC, biochemistry panel, coagulation panel or ACT, CXR (enlarged, globoid cardiac silhouette with small pulmonary vessels +/− pleural effusion). The globoid cardiac silhouette must be differentiated from dilated cardiomyopathy, which has an enlarged heart with large pulmonary vessels +/− pulmonary edema. An echocardiogram should be done (pericardial effusion +/− tamponade; collapse of the right heart, +/− mass). Ideally perform an echocardiogram BEFORE pericardiocentesis to optimize visualization of masses. Do not delay pericardiocentesis if unstable.

Treatment

- Pericardiocentesis
  See "Pericardial effusion" section later for procedure.
- Initiate crystalloid fluids (@ 1.5–2.0 × maintenance rate if stable; larger volumes may be required in unstable patients).
  Furosemide is contraindicated.

 Prognosis

With idiopathic pericardial effusion approximately 50% will need repeated taps. Definitive treatment is surgery (pericardiectomy). With hemangiosarcoma the prognosis is poor and life span is 1 to 4 months depending on metastasis and treatment options chosen. Other tumors tend to be slower growing and the prognosis is guarded to poor. Good prognosis if secondary to anticoagulant rodenticide.

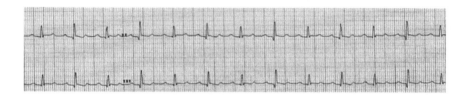

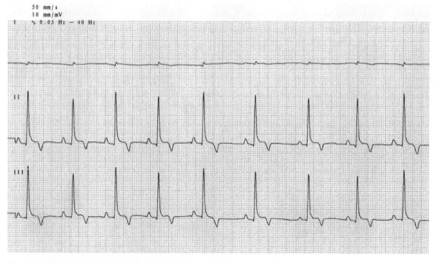

Figures 57 and 58 Electrical alternans.

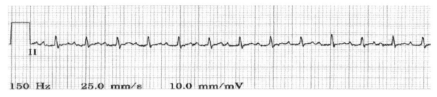

150 Hz   25.0 mm/s   10.0 mm/mV

Figure 59 Low-amplitude QRS.

Left bundle branch block

 ## Recognition

In most cases a P wave occurs before every QRS (activation is occurring from above the ventricle), QRS greater than 0.08 s in dogs and 0.06 s in cats (wide), the R wave is upright in lead I, II, III and aVF, and the P-R interval is normal. Left axis deviation may occur.

 ## Differentials and diagnostics

Bundle branch block is indicative of interruption of conduction through the bundle of His and may be paroxysmal (intermittent) or continuous. When an impulse travels towards the ventricle the blocked branch is activated later than the unblocked branch leading to asynchronous activation of the ventricles. This leads to a widening of the QRS. It may indicate cardiac hypertrophy and can easily be misinterpreted as a ventricular arrhythmia.

 ## Treatment

This is an uncommon rhythm. Bundle branch blocks do not directly impair cardiac function. The underlying cause should be addressed (e.g., cardiac consult).

 ## Prognosis

Guarded.

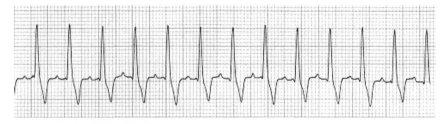

Figure 60 Left bundle branch block.

Left anterior fascicular block

 Recognition

Tall R wave in lead I and aVL, deep S wave in leads II, III, aVF. Left axis deviation. QRS is of normal duration.

 Differentials and diagnostics

The left anterior fascicle is a subdivision of the left bundle branch. This arrhythmia indicates a block in the left anterior fascicle of the left bundle branch (LAFB) causing delayed depolarization of the left ventricle. LAFB is common in cats and may be associated with hypertrophic cardiomyopathy (HCM). It may also be seen with ischemic conditions or hyperkalemia.

 Treatment

This arrhythmia does not directly impair cardiac function so no specific treatment indicated but cardiac workup should be considered.

 Prognosis

Guarded depending on cause or underlying disease.

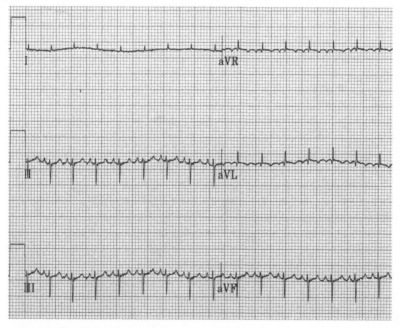

Figure 61 Left anterior fascicular block.

Right bundle branch block

 Recognition

In most cases a P wave occurs before every QRS (activation is occurring from above the ventricle), QRS greater than 0.08 s in dogs and 0.06 s in cats (wide), the R wave is negative in lead II, there are large, wide S waves in leads I, II, III and aVF, and the P-R interval is normal. Right axis deviation is seen.

 Differentials and diagnostics

Bundle branch block is indicative of interruption of conduction through the bundle of His and may be paroxysmal (intermittent) or continuous. When an impulse travels towards the ventricle the blocked branch is activated later than the unblocked branch leading to asynchronous activation of the ventricles. This leads to a widening of the QRS. It may indicate cardiac hypertrophy and can easily be misinterpreted as a ventricular arrhythmia. Rule outs include heartworm disease, pulmonary thromboembolism, Chagas cardiomyopathy, neoplasia, and hyperkalemia.

 Treatment

No specific treatment indicated for arrhythmia but cardiac workup should be considered along with a heartworm test and, if indicated, testing for Chagas disease.

 Prognosis

Guarded.

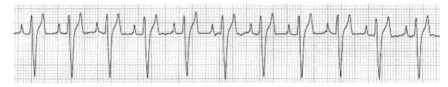

Figure 62 Right bundle branch block.

ST segment abnormalities

 Recognition

The ST segment can be elevated or depressed from baseline.

Differentials and diagnostics

The ST segment is the time from the end of the QRS to the onset of the T wave and indicates the early phase of ventricular repolarization. Elevation may indicate myocardial hypoxia, infarct, or pericarditis. Depression may indicate myocardial hypoxia, infarct, trauma, digoxin toxicity, or alterations in serum potassium.

 Treatment

Treat the underlying cause.

 Prognosis

Guarded.

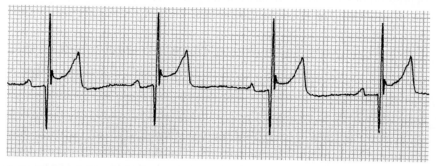

Figure 63 ST segment elevation.

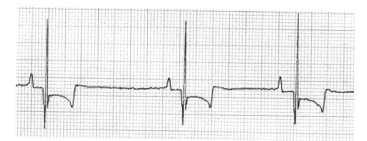

Figure 64 ST segment depression.

T wave abnormalities

 Recognition

The normal T wave represents repolarization of the ventricles and is the first major deflection after the QRS. It can be positive (upright), negative (downward), notched, or biphasic. It should be ≤25% of the R wave height and should retain the same shape (not change from negative to positive) during evaluation.

 Differentials and diagnostics

Tall tented (sharp) T waves: Hyperkalemia is the first consideration. Other ECG changes associated with hyperkalemia are small to absent P wave, a regular rhythm (constant R-R intervals) and usually (not always) bradycardia. Bradycardia may not be present or may not be recognized if T wave approaches R wave height. The ECG will read tallest wave as R wave to count and may provide a double count for the heart rate (e.g., cat with HR 200 bpm on ECG may actually be 100 bpm on auscultation). Eventually widening of QRS, ventricular fibrillation and asystole occur.
- Depression or elevation from baseline may indicate myocardial hypoxia, cardiac hypertrophy, or electrolyte alterations. Electrolytes and cardiac consult are recommended.
- Low amplitude or inverted T waves may indicate hypokalemia, hypocalcemia, or ischemia.

 Treatment

Calcium gluconate 10% at 0.5–1.5 mL/kg slow IV over 20–30 min while monitoring the ECG. This provides "cardioprotection" but does not decrease potassium concentration. Definitive treatment for hyperkalemia should occur ASAP (e.g., urethral obstruction, uroabdomen, acute renal failure, hypoadrenocorticism, and so on). Refer to emergency texts for treatment of these underlying causes.

 Prognosis

Guarded.

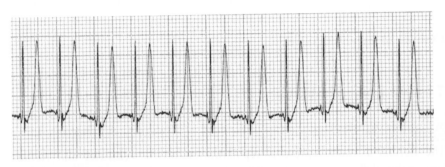

Figure 65 Enlarged T wave.

Canine congestive heart failure—mitral valve insufficiency

 Recognition

The classic mitral regurgitation (MR) patient is an older, small breed dog. Often there is a history of increased respiratory rate and cough, which may be worse at night, and the dog may be uncomfortable lying down. May see weight loss, decreased appetite, or syncope. Smaller breeds may have concurrent tracheal collapse. Ask dietary history (stable MR dog may decompensate with a high salt diet). Cough, tachypnea, dyspnea, pale to cyanotic mucous membranes, weak pulses, heart murmur +/− gallop rhythm, +/− ascites, weakness, cachexia, may hear crackles on thoracic auscultation.

 Differentials and diagnostics

Auscultation may reveal crackles or wheezes, increased broncho-vesicular sounds, or may be normal. Pulse oximetry may be abnormal (less than 98% saturation), ideally a minimum data base (PCV, TS, azo, BG), electrolytes, and CBC and biochemistry panel are submitted but many animals are not stable enough for this. If dog is stable consider ECG (normal or wide, notched P wave indicating LA enlargement), CXR (cardiomegaly, pulmonary edema, +/− compression of the left main-stem bronchus), echocardiogram (mitral regurgitation), blood pressure, and UA for baseline renal function. If not stable, proceed to the treatment section (below).

 Treatment

- Oxygen by least stressful method.
- Furosemide (2–4 mg/kg IV or IM, then 1–2 mg/kg q15min to 1 h as needed), or furosemide CRI (0.5–1.0 mg/kg/h) until respiratory rate decreases by half. Then decrease to 2 mg/kg q6–8h. Strict cage rest, walk only in ICU, free choice water at all times.
- Consider butorphanol (0.2–0.4 mg/kg IV or IM), or midazolam (0.05–0.1 mg/kg IM) for anxiety.
- If ascites is severe and impinging respiration, abdominocentesis. If patient is unstable remove only enough to make comfortable; if patient is stable remove as much as possible.
- IV fluids with CHF is contraindicated but if severely azotemic, may need to consider concurrent IV fluids (plasmalyte 56 or 0.45% NaCl in 2.5% dextrose or Normosol-M) @ $1/4$ to $1/2$ maintenance rate. Not an ideal situation, prognosis guarded.

- Apply nitroglycerin paste 2% ($^1/_4$ to $^1/_2$ inch applied to clipped area on thorax or ear pinnae, cover and label).
- Dyspnea

    If severe, acute, unresponsive dyspnea in animal with previous history of MR consider LA rupture or rupture of chordae tendinae. This can be diagnosed on echocardiogram.

    - Consider sodium nitroprusside @ 0.5–3.0 µg/kg/min IV CRI. Start at low dose and titrate up q15–30min depending on clinical response. Monitor blood pressure as severe hypotension can result. Stop nitroprusside when MAP ≤ 60 mmHg or systolic blood pressure is < 90 mmHg. Drug is light sensitive—cover line and bag. Cyanide toxicity may occur if overdose or rapid bolus—label line and catheter "DO NOT FLUSH."

 Prognosis

Good for short term with mild clinical signs, guarded to poor for long term or if concurrent azotemia. Poor with severe clinical signs or ruptured chordae or LA.

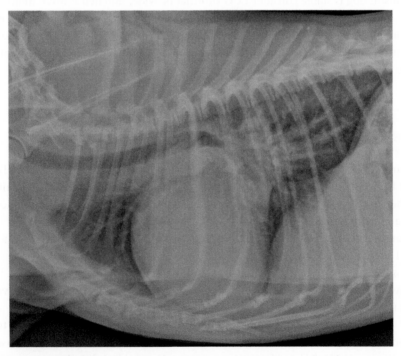

Figures 66 and 67 Thoracic radiographs of congestive heart failure.

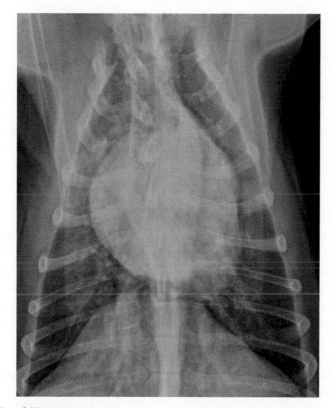

Figures 66 and 67 (*Continued*)

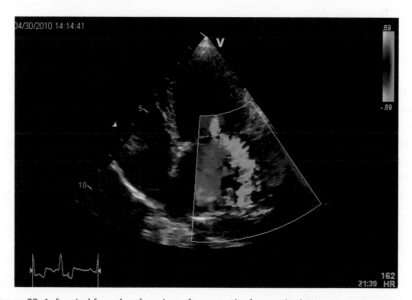

Figure 68 Left apical four chamber view of severe mitral regurgitation.

Canine dilated cardiomyopathy

 Recognition

Generally a giant/large breed dog or a Cocker Spaniel. May have history of weakness, exercise intolerance, syncope, or tachypnea. May have weak pulses, pale or cyanotic mucous membranes, hypothermia, cold extremities due to inadequate cardiac output (cardiogenic shock). Animal may also have pleural effusion, ascites, pulmonary edema, and atrial fibrillation (rapid, chaotic heartbeat with pulse deficits). See "Atrial fibrillation" section in Chapter 3.

 Differentials and diagnostics

Auscultation may reveal quiet lung sounds (pleural effusion) or rapid, chaotic heart sounds with pulse deficits (atrial fibrillation). Pulse oximetry may be abnormal (less than 98% saturation), ideally a minimum data base (PCV, TS, azo, BG), electrolytes, and CBC, and biochemistry panel are submitted but many animals are not stable enough for this. If stable consider ECG (tachycardia with irregularly irregular rhythm, and no visible P waves; see "Atrial fibrillation" section in Chapter 3), CXR (generalized cardiomegaly, pleural effusion, or pulmonary edema), echocardiogram (decreased contractility), blood pressure, and UA for baseline renal function. Consider submitting blood for taurine levels. If the animal is not stable, proceed to the treatment section.

 Treatment

- Minimize stress
- Oxygen supplementation
- IV catheter when stable
- Taurine (250 mg orally q12h) and L-carnitine (100 mg/kg orally q8h) if Cocker Spaniel.
- For atrial fibrillation can slow ventricular rate if HR > 180 bpm and affecting perfusion (urine output, lactate, extremity temperature, pulse quality, mentation) with diltiazem @ 0.25 mg/kg IV over 10 min through a peripheral vein, followed by a CRI @ 1–5 μg/kg/min.
  - *Or* procainamide (15 mg/kg IV over 10 min, to effect), follow with a CRI @ 25–50 μg/kg/min.
  - Begin digoxin (0.005–0.008 mg/kg/day orally divided q12h) and check levels in 5–7 days.
  - Add beta blocker if no response: propranolol (0.2–1 mg/kg orally q8h) or sotalol (1–2 mg/kg orally q12h), beta blockers are contraindicated if there is pulmonary edema.

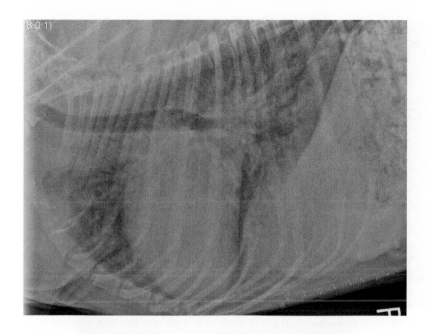

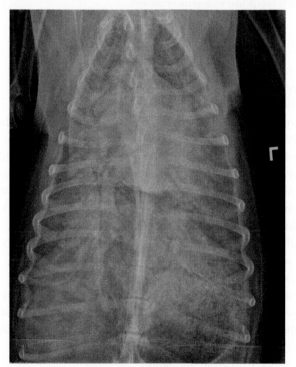

Figures 69 and 70 Thoracic radiographs of a dog with DCM and congestive heart failure.

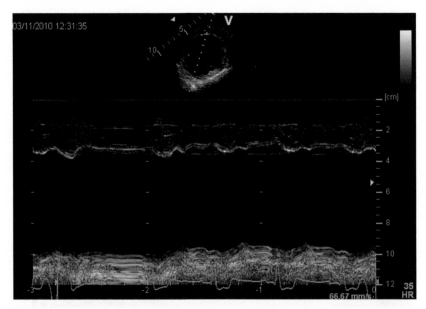

Figure 71 Right parasternal short axis M-mode view of left ventricle. Severe systolic dsyfunction and left ventricular enlargement present.

- Pulmonary edema

  If pulmonary edema present give furosemide (2–4 mg/kg IV, IM).
- Pleural effusion

  Perform thoracocentesis. Administer sedation if necessary (butorphanol 0.2 mg/kg IV, IM, SC). Sterile prep of 7–9th ICS (ventrally). For small dogs attach butterfly catheter or 22 g one-inch needle or over-the-needle catheter to three-way stopcock and 12–20 mL syringe; for larger dogs attach 18–22 g one or one and a half-inch needle or OTN catheter to three-way stopcock and 35–60 mL syringe. Insert needle perpendicular to chest, have someone aspirate syringe and as soon as tap is positive, non-traumatically aim needle caudo-laterally. Remove as much fluid as possible (except with hemorrhagic effusions) and stop when get negative tap or blood in syringe.
- Cardiogenic shock without atrial fibrillation

  Use dobutamine (5 μg/kg/min IV CRI), increase by 2 μg/kg/min q15min to effect (increased urine output, warm extremities, stronger pulses) or until HR > 200 bpm or cardiac arrhythmias develop, worsen or animal vomits. If necessary restart in 30 min, decrease dose by 20–30%.
- Cardiogenic shock with atrial fibrillation

  Reduce ventricular response rate first with diltiazem (0.25 mg/kg IV over 10 min). Can repeat 2 times. If rate comes down and cardiogenic shock still present (weak pulses, no urine, cold extremities) can add dobutamine. Do

not give dobutamine to dog in atrial fibrillation without diltiazem first. Dobutamine increases ventricular response to atrial fibrillation and can cause fatal
arrhythmia.

- Pulmonary edema and cardiogenic shock
Start dobutamine first, then add sodium nitroprusside @ 0.5–3 μg/kg/min
IV CRI. Start at low dose and titrate up q15–30min depending on clinical
response. Monitor blood pressure as severe hypotension can result. Stop nitroprusside when MAP ≤ 60 mmHg or systolic blood pressure is < 90 mmHg. Drug
is light sensitive—cover line and bag. Cyanide toxicity if overdose or rapid
bolus—label line and catheter "DO NOT FLUSH."

 Prognosis

Poor for long term, guarded to poor for short term.

Feline aortic thromboembolism (saddle thrombus)

 Recognition

Peracute onset of paralysis or paresis of both hind limbs, one hind limb, or
one forelimb. May have a history of possible trauma (outdoor cat comes home
dragging hind limbs and owner assumes trauma). The affected limb or limbs are
usually cold and painful. There are often absent or weak pulses, and pale or
cyanotic footpads and nail beds. The rectal temperature may be decreased and
male cats may be predisposed. Many have no history of cardiomyopathy.

 Differentials and diagnostics

Must rule out trauma, especially in outdoor cats with unknown history. Consider
thoracic radiographs (pulmonary edema, pleural effusion), spinal radiographs
(fracture of pelvis, spine, etc.), ECG, echocardiogram (underlying cardiomyopathy, smoke in left atrium, clot in left atrium), CBC and biochemistry panel to
rule out comorbid conditions. The coagulation panel is often unrewarding as PT
and aPTT cannot be used to indicate a pro-thrombotic state. This condition can be
very painful and it is imperative to differentiate the cause of tachypnea (pain ver-
sus pulmonary edema/pleural effusion) as furosemide may be indicated in addi-
tion to analgesia. Blood from the affected limb will often be lower in blood glu-
cose and higher in lactate compared to blood from a central vein due to decreased
perfusion and this can be helpful to help differentiate thromboembolism from
trauma.

Treatment

Consists of some combination of oxygen, analgesia, furosemide, unfractionated or low molecular weight heparin, physical therapy, antiplatelet agents (e.g., aspirin, clopidogrel) depending on other conditions (e.g., congestive heart failure, smoke in left atrium, and so on). Thrombolytic agents can cause life-threatening complications and should only be administered with caution.

- Oxygen by least stressful method until pulmonary edema or pleural effusion are ruled out.
- Analgesia options include butorphanol at 0.2–0.4 mg/kg IV, IM, or fentanyl at 2–6 μg/kg IV, or methadone at 0.05–0.5 mg/kg IV, IM, SC q4h. Analgesia is essential as this is a very painful condition.
- Furosemide at 2–4 mg/kg IV or IM q4–8h if indicated.
- Unfractionated heparin @ 150 U/kg SC q8h will not dissolve the clot but may prevent new clots from forming.
- *Or* Low molecular weight heparin. Options include dalteparin (Fragmin®) at 150 U/kg SC q6h to q8h or enoxaparin (Lovenox®) at 1.5 mg/kg SC q8h. Dosages are unclear—there are no definitive dosages proven to work in cats with pro-thrombotic conditions. This will not dissolve the clot but may prevent new clots from forming.
- Aspirin can be started 36–48 h before stopping heparin at 1.0 mg/kg PO q24h. An 81 mg aspirin can be crushed and placed into a syringe with 10 mL tap water and thoroughly shaken. Each mL will be ~8 mg and the owner can discard the rest after giving the appropriate dose each day.
- *Or* clopidogrel (Plavix®) can be started 36–48 h before stopping heparin at 18.75 mg/cat PO q24h. This will not dissolve the clot but may prevent new clots from forming.
- Physical therapy should be started as soon as the cat is stable. Keep the limbs warm (e.g., no electric heating pads, cats are predisposed to burns due to lack of sensation in the hypo-perfused limbs).
- Thrombolytics have a very high rate of life-threatening complications and their use is often discouraged. Streptokinase at 90,000 units IV over 4 h, followed by 45,000 units per hour for 3 h has been reported to dissolve clots. Bradycardia and hyperkalemia are frequently reported side effects (from reperfusion injury) and ECG and electrolyte monitoring are essential. Bleeding from catheter or injection sites is also common and the cat may need a blood transfusion if severe bleeding occurs. If bleeding occurs there is minimal benefit to vitamin K1 therapy as it takes ~8–12 h to work and will interfere with some anti-coagulant treatments for ~1 week. For hyperkalemia causing bradycardia give 10% calcium gluconate at 0.5–1.0 mL/kg slow IV over 20 min. If the cat does not have pulmonary edema or pleural effusion consider crystalloid fluids (0.9% NaCl at 5 mL/kg bolus) to decrease potassium. If hyperkalemia persists

consider dextrose bolus or regular insulin with dextrose to move potassium intracellularly.

 Prognosis

Guarded for return of function, poor for long term.

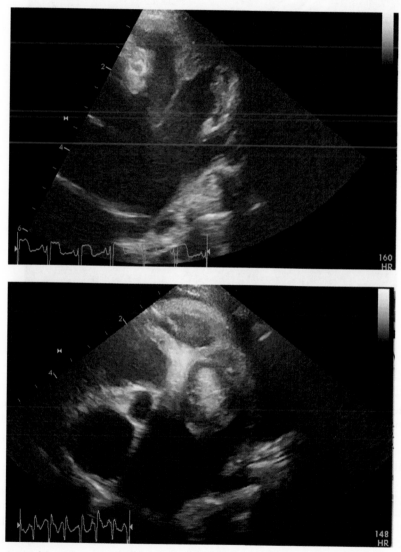

Figures 72–73 Left cranial short axis view of the left atrium and left auricle. There is a large thrombus present in the tip of the auricle.

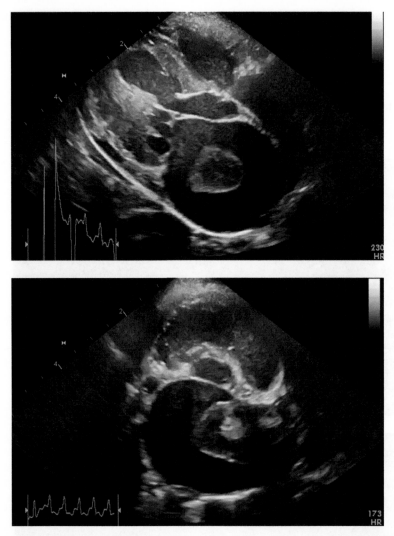

Figures 74–75 Right parasternal long axis view of a ball thrombus in the left atrium. Right parasternal short axis of the left atrium and aorta showing a large mural thrombus in the left atrium and auricle.

Feline congestive heart failure

 Recognition

Respiratory distress, may occur suddenly with no prior history of cardiac disease. Alternatively, may have a history of HCM, DCM, or RCM. Pale or cyanotic mucous membranes, prolonged CRT, tachypnea, normal to increased bronchovesicular lung sounds, crackles/wheezes or quiet lungs sounds (pleural effusion) may be present as well as heart murmur or gallop rhythm with weak pulses.

Differentials and diagnostics

Cats with pulmonary edema may have normal lung sounds, may or may not have heart murmur or gallop rhythm, and are often hypothermic. Must differentiate from other causes of respiratory distress (e.g., trauma, asthma, pyothorax). Asthma may cause increased broncho-vesicular sounds or crackles or wheezes and may have a prolonged expiratory phase. Thoracic radiographs may be diagnostic but should only be done when the cat is stable. Pulmonary edema may manifest as a patchy alveolar pattern, a diffuse alveolar pattern, a broncho-interstitial pattern, or numerous combination patterns in cats so may be more difficult to diagnose than in dogs. The ECG will often be normal and the echocardiogram can be useful to diagnose cardiomyopathy but should only be done when the cat is stable. The minimum data base, CBC, biochemistry panel, FeLV/FIV, heartworm test, and urinalysis are all helpful to rule out concurrent or underlying conditions.

 Treatment

- Oxygen by least stressful method (usually cage or incubator) while assessing and preparing supplies.
- Thoracocentesis is both diagnostic and therapeutic and should be performed if tachypnea (with shallow breathing/quiet lung sounds) is present.
  - Perform thoracocentesis
    Administer sedation if necessary (butorphanol 0.2 mg/kg IV, IM, SC). This is rarely needed. Sterile prep of 7–9th ICS (latero-ventrally). Attach butterfly catheter or 22 g one-inch needle or over-the-needle catheter to three-way stopcock and 6–12 mL syringe. Insert needle perpendicular to chest, have someone aspirate syringe and as soon as tap is positive, non-traumatically aim needle caudo-laterally. Remove as much fluid as possible (except with hemorrhagic effusions) and stop when get negative tap or blood in syringe.
- Rapid placement of IV catheter if possible, give injections IM if too stressful.
- Furosemide at 2 mg/kg IV, IM, may repeat q2–4h. In some cases repeating the first dose 30 min later is necessary.
- Dobutamine can be used in cats with hypotension and low output heart failure, significant hypoperfusion, or are not responding adequately to aggressive diuretic therapy. Doses of 2–10 μg/kg/min are typically used, starting at this low end and increasing slowly until effective.
- Nitroglycerin paste 1/4 to 1/2 inch applied to clipped area on thorax or pinnae, cover and label.
- Sodium nitroprusside
  If no improvement after repeated doses of furosemide, oxygen, +/− thoracocentesis attempt, and blood pressure is normal, consider sodium nitroprusside. This is given at 0.5–3.0 μg/kg/min. Start low, titrate up q15min depending on

clinical response. Monitor blood pressure as this can cause severe hypotension. DO NOT FLUSH IV catheter and be sure to label IV catheter "Do Not Flush." Stop drug if hypotension develops.

 Prognosis

Guarded to poor for long term.

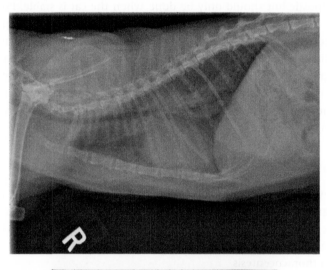

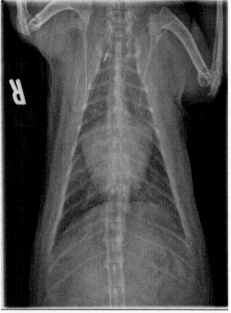

Figures 76–79 2 view thoracic radiographs of a cat with severe cardiac enlargement, perihilar pulmonary edema, and venous congestion.

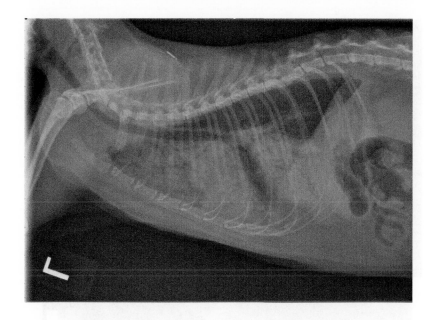

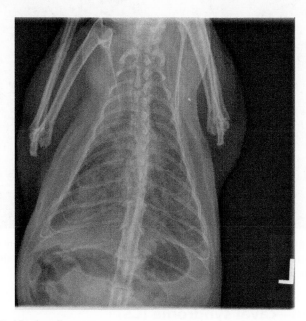

Figures 76–79 (*Continued*)

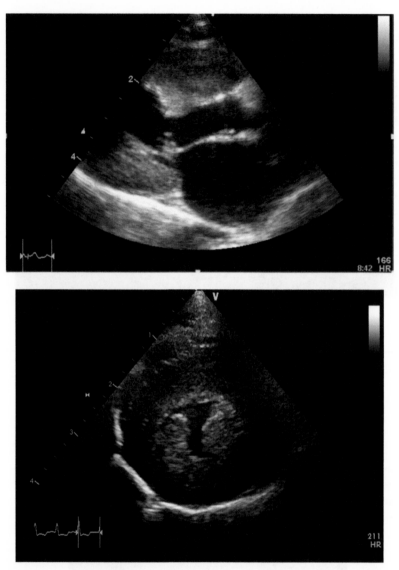

Figures 80 and 81 Right parasternal long axis view showing severe left atrial enlargement and left ventricular concentric hypertrophy. Right parasternal short axis view of the left ventricle showing severe left ventricular concentric hypertrophy.

Heartworm—caval syndrome (CS)

 Recognition

From right heart failure due to mass of heartworms in right atrium, right ventricle, vena cava, or main pulmonary artery. Often dog has a large worm burden and significant pulmonary artery disease (pulmonary hypertension). May have a history of cough, exercise intolerance, weakness, and hemoptysis. On physical examination there may be weakness, jugular vein distension, jugular pulses, weak peripheral pulses, pale mucous membranes, tachypnea, harsh lung sounds, pleural effusion, icterus, enlarged liver, ascites, and hemoglobinuria. A systolic heart murmur (tricuspid insufficiency) and a loud, split S2 may be auscultated.

 ## Differentials and diagnostics

If the animal is stable collect for a minimum data base (PCV, TS, azo, BG), CBC (may see anemia, hemoglobinemia, thrombocytopenia, eosinophilia +/− basophilia, may see microfilaria), biochemistry panel (may see elevated liver enzymes, hyperglobulinemia), and heartworm test. Also consider an ECG (may see right shift of mean electrical axis), coagulation panel, UA (may see hemoglobinuria). An echocardiogram should be done as soon as possible to visualize the worms. It may identify a large number of worms moving from RA to RV. Thoracic radiographs may reveal tortuous, blunted pulmonary arteries, enlarged main pulmonary artery segment, right-sided cardiomegaly, patchy alveolar infiltrates, pleural effusion, and pulmonary edema.

 ## Treatment

- Oxygen supplementation by the least stressful method (flow by or cage).
- If suspect caval syndrome place peripheral catheter; **do not use jugular veins** (save for surgical removal of worms).
- Surgical removal of heartworms as soon as possible. See below.
- IV fluids with 0.45% NaCl and 2.5% dextrose (start at $^1/_2$ maintenance rate).
- Consider anti-inflammatory dose of corticosteroids (prednisone @ 0.5 mg/kg PO or dexamethasone @ 0.05 mg/kg IV).
- Thoracocentesis if pleural effusion present.
- Abdominocentesis if ascites compromises respiration, only remove enough to make dog comfortable.
- Remove worms; in many dogs this can be performed under sedation; however, general anesthesia is often required. This procedure should be performed using fluoroscopy. Aseptically prep right ventro-lateral neck and infiltrate with lidocaine.
  - Surgery
    Make incision to isolate the jugular vein and ligate it cranial to intended entry. Make a small incision in jugular vein, insert basket retrieval device or Ishihara forceps into the right atrium and right ventricle to remove worms. Care should be taken not to rupture worms or inadvertently damage cardiac structures (tricuspid valve). When several attempts come up empty

and no worms are visualized on echocardiogram, ligate jugular vein, suture incision.

- Monitor closely during recovery, oxygen supplementation, low stress, monitor blood pressure, pulse oximetry, Hct/TS, lactate, electrolytes, and arterial blood gas. Patients are at high risk for multi-organ system failure, systemic inflammatory response syndrome, and disseminated intravascular coagulation (DIC).
- Consider Plavix (clopidogrel) 1–2 mg/kg q24h and prednisone (0.5 mg/kg q24h for 1 week, then 0.25 mg/kg q24h for 1 week).
- If right-sided heart failure consider furosemide (2 mg/kg IV, IM q12h, pimobendan 0.25–0.35 mg/kg PO q12h, and sildenafil 2–3 mg/kg PO q12h.
- If stable, send home on strict cage rest for 2–4 weeks before considering adulticide treatments. Start doxycycline (10 mg/kg PO q12h) to suppress infection/inflammation from Wolbachia bacteria.
- If worms not retrievable consider treatment with adulticide, melarsomine @ 2.5 mg/kg deep IM once, then repeat in 1 month for two additional treatments 24 h apart. Many dogs will not tolerate adulticide therapy if they have a large worm burden within their right atrium and ventricle and are at high risk for fatal thromboembolism if treatment is given.
- Microfilaricide can be administered 3–4 weeks after completion of adulticide treatment.
  - Anaphylaxis can occur, often within 2–4 h of giving oral dose. Most likely related to death of large amounts of microfilaria. Treat for anaphylaxis with oxygen, shock dose of crystalloids, and colloids as follows:
    Administer isotonic crystalloid bolus:
    Dogs: 20 mL/kg (up to 90 mL/kg); Cats: 10 mL/kg (up to 45 mL/kg) and then reassess perfusion.
    If minimal improvement consider synthetic colloids (HES):
    Dogs: 5 mL/kg bolus over 15–20 min and reassess perfusion. Give up to 20 mL/kg total.
    Cats: 2–5 mL/kg bolus over 20–30 min and reassess perfusion. Do not bolus colloids rapidly to cats. Give up to 10 mL/kg total.
  - Also administer dexamethasone (0.05 mg/kg IV), diphenhydramine (1–2 mg/kg IM), and consider epinephrine (0.01 mg/kg IV, IM).
- Monitor MAP, continuous ECG, CVP, pulse oximetry, urine output, lactate, electrolytes, PCV, TS. Continue fluid support to maintain systolic BP > 90 mmHg.

 Prognosis

Poor if DIC, BUN > 60 and/or increased ALT, guarded if no evidence of DIC, BUN < 60.

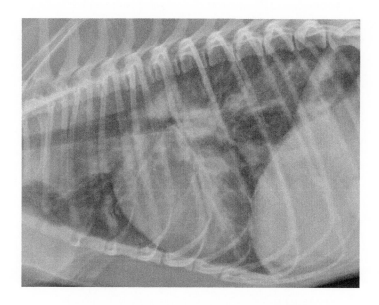

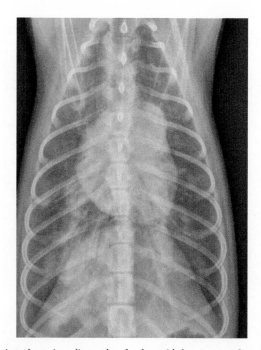

Figures 82–85 2 view thoracic radiographs of a dog with heartworm disease. Note patchy interstitial-alveolar lung pattern consistent with pneumonitis. The pulmonary arteries are moderately to severely enlarged and there is right ventricular enlargement noted by the "reverse D" on the VD views.

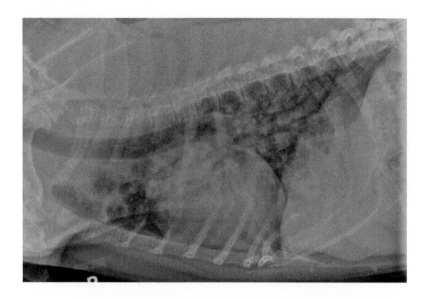

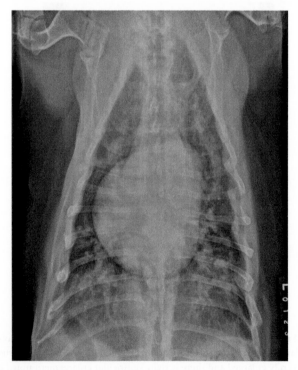

Figures 82–85 (*Continued*)

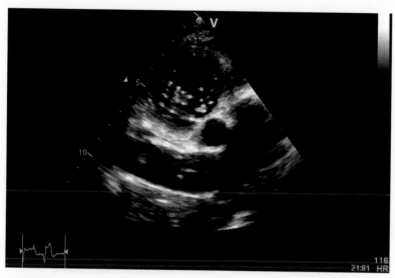

Figure 86 Right parasternal short axis view of the pulmonary artery, aorta, and right atrium. Note the hyperechoic parallel lines (adult heartworms) in the right atrium as well as the right branch pulmonary artery.

Pericardial effusion

 Recognition

The history may include weakness, exercise intolerance, collapse, polyuria, poly-dipsia, vomiting. German Shepherd and Golden Retriever dogs are predisposed. Approximately 19% are idiopathic and 59% are neoplastic. Occasionally see other causes such as coagulopathy (anticoagulant rodenticide), ruptured LA, infectious disease, biventricular failure. On physical examination the animal may be weak and have pale to cyanotic mucous membranes, jugular venous distention +/− jugular pulses, muffled heart sounds, weak pulses, pulsus paradoxicus (weaker pulses on inspiration), tachycardia.

 Differentials and diagnostics

ECG (electrical alternans is a variation in the height of the R wave with every other beat, small QRS complexes with R wave <1 mV), minimum data base (PCV, TS, azo, BG), CBC, biochemistry panel, coagulation panel or ACT, thoracic radio-graphs (may see enlarged, globoid cardiac silhouette with small pulmonary vessels +/− pleural effusion). This must be differentiated from dilated cardiomyopa-thy, which has an enlarged heart with large pulmonary vessels +/− pulmonary edema. An echocardiogram should be done (should see pericardial effusion +/− tamponade; collapse of the right heart, +/− mass). Ideally perform an echocar-diogram BEFORE pericardiocentesis to optimize visualization of masses. Do not delay pericardiocentesis if unstable.

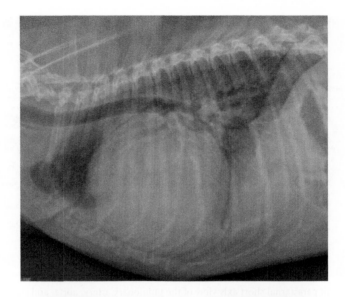

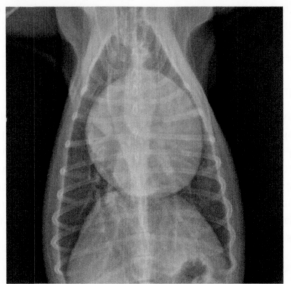

Figures 87 and 88 Thoracic radiograph. Note globoid cardiac silhouette.

 Treatment

- Pericardiocentesis
  - Monitor ECG during entire procedure.
  - Sterile prep right side of chest (avoid coronary vessels on left).
  - Local block

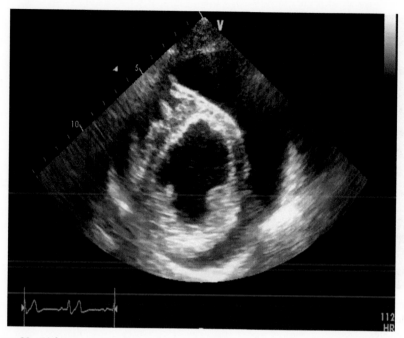

Figure 89   Right parasternal short axis view of the left ventricle. Note the surrounding anechoic fluid consistent with severe pericardial effusion.

Infuse 0.9 mL lidocaine combined with 0.1 mL sodium bicarbonate to the right 4–5 ICS at the level of the costochondral junction (CCJ).

- Prepare a 35 mL (medium-sized dog) or 60 mL (large dog) syringe attached to a three-way stopcock, extension tubing, and a 14–16 g venocath.
- Pericardiocentesis
  Slowly enter the chest at the 4–5 ICS at the level of the CC junction (with the stopcock turned off to patient). Advance catheter into chest and turn the stopcock on to patient (off to open port or outside), put negative pressure on syringe. A pop is often felt when the pericardium is entered and fluid will begin to enter the syringe. Advance the catheter 1.0 cm while holding the stylet steady, keep system in place to empty pericardial sac. Alternatively, can remove the stylet to avoid the needle causing damage to structures and reconnect the extension tubing for suctioning and emptying of the sac.
- Coagulopathy
  Ideally a PT or aPTT or ACT should be done before pericardiocentesis especially in at-risk dogs (e.g., young dog, farm dog, and so on). If there are other signs of coagulation defects (e.g., bleeding from IV catheter site, bleeding from venipuncture sites) be sure to get a PT or aPTT or ACT before pericardiocentesis.
- As soon as the first syringe is full replace it and with the effusion in the syringe measure the HCT/TS on the fluid and check that it does not clot. (It should not

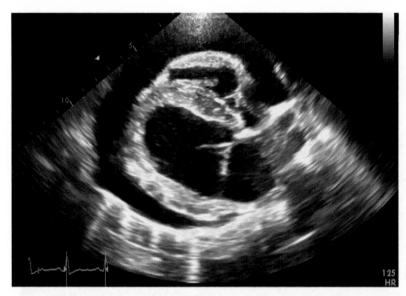

Figure 90 Echocardiogram of PE. Right parasternal long axis view of severe pericardial effusion. Note the collapse of the right atrium at the top of image consistent with cardiac tamponade.

clot, clotting may indicate you are in the heart itself.) The HCT should be a bit lower than the peripheral HCT (an equal HCT might indicate you are in the heart).

- Submit samples for fluid analysis, cytology, C&S.
- Remove as much as possible while monitoring the ECG for arrhythmias (if arrhythmias develop it may indicate catheter touching myocardium, partially withdraw needle and reassess).

  Occasionally only a small amount of fluid is recovered when effusion leaks out of the pericardium into the thoracic cavity. If this is the case, clinically the animal will improve dramatically despite the small amount of fluid retrieved.

- Initiate crystalloid fluids (@ 1.5–2.0 × maintenance rate if stable, larger volumes may be required in unstable patients).

  Furosemide is contraindicated.

 Prognosis

With idiopathic PE approximately 50% will need repeated taps. Definitive treatment is surgery (pericardectomy). With hemangiosarcoma the prognosis is poor and life span is 1 to 4 months depending on metastasis and treatment options. Other tumors tend to be slower growing and the prognosis is guarded to poor. Good prognosis if secondary to anticoagulant rodenticide.

Chapter 5 Electrolyte disturbance and the ECG

Hyperkalemia

 Recognition

Depending on the degree of hyperkalemia (the potassium concentration) and the individual animal, any or all of the following may be seen: small or absent P wave in all leads, tall and tented (sharp or pointed) T wave, small QRS, widening of QRS, bradycardia, ventricular fibrillation, asystole. When the T wave approaches the height of the R wave the ECG monitor may double count as it counts the tallest wave as an R wave. This can lead to the mis-diagnosis of ventricular tachycardia and MUST be verified with auscultation before treatment for tachycardia is instituted.

 Differentials and diagnostics

Most commonly caused by urinary obstruction (cats > dogs), urinary tract rupture (uroabdomen), hypoadrenocorticism, acute kidney injury, acute tumor lysis syndrome, reperfusion injury, toxicity, and others.

 Treatment

Emergency treatment for hyperkalemia that is affecting the heart (ECG changes) is calcium gluconate 10% slow IV at 0.5–1.5 mL/kg over 20–30 min. Always monitor with ECG and if there is a sudden decrease in HR stop infusion. Never exceed 10 mL of calcium gluconate as a bolus. This will afford a short period of cardioprotection (~20 min) while the specific condition is addressed. Calcium gluconate does not reduce the serum potassium concentration. Address the underlying issue.

 Prognosis

Guarded.

Life-Threatening Cardiac Emergencies for the Small Animal Practitioner, First Edition. Maureen McMichael and Ryan Fries.
© 2016 John Wiley & Sons, Inc. Published 2016 by John Wiley & Sons, Inc.

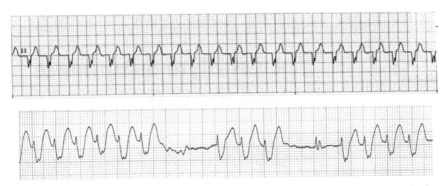

Figures 91 and 92 Hyperkalemia. Note the wide QRS complexes, tall T waves, and lack of P waves. *Source*: Figure 91 courtesy of Gregg Rapoport.

Hypokalemia

 Recognition

Ventricular premature contractions may be present. Other ECG changes may include progressive flattening of the T wave, ST segment depression, wide T wave (called a U wave), and a prolonged QT interval. Other clinical signs that may be present include muscle weakness, ventroflexion of the neck, renal, and gastrointestinal signs.

 Differentials and diagnostics

Generally a workup to include CBC, biochemistry panel, urinalysis, etc. is indicated to rule out numerous causes.

 Treatment

Potassium chloride (KCL) supplementation orally or IV according to potassium supplement charts. Do not exceed 0.5 mEq/kg/h of KCL.

 Prognosis

Guarded.

Hypercalcemia

 Recognition

Short QT interval, normal T wave. Other signs of hypercalcemia include polyuria and polydipsia, weakness, and others specific to underlying cause (e.g., neoplasia).

Differentials and diagnostics

Possibilities include vitamin D toxicity (rodenticides, human psoriasis creams, human medications or vitamins), lymphoma, chronic kidney disease, hypoa-drenocorticism, apocrine gland adenocarcinoma, primary hypoparathyroidism, multiple myeloma, and others.

 Treatment

Calcium-free crystalloid fluids, furosemide. See an emergency or internal medicine textbook for detailed treatment guidelines.

 Prognosis

Guarded.

Hypocalcemia

 Recognition

A prolonged QT interval, normal T wave, may have tachycardia. Other signs of hypocalcemia are muscle fasciculations (tremors), hyperthermia, panting, facial rubbing, stiff gait, seizures, and elevated nictitating membranes in cats.

 Differentials and diagnostics

Lab error (always check), eclampsia (history and physical will reveal a lactating female), hypoparathyroidism, ethylene glycol toxicity (low ionized calcium, oxalate crystals seen on urinalysis), pancreatitis (saponification causing calcium-phosphorous complex formation).

 Treatment

Calcium gluconate 10% at 0.5–1.5 mL/kg IV over 20–30 min (do not exceed 10 mL per bolus). The goal is to alleviate clinical signs and address the underlying condition, not to bring the calcium back to the normal range immediately.

 Prognosis

Guarded.

Chapter 6 Emergency algorithms

Bradycardia algorithm

An algorithm to follow for diagnosis and treatment of significant bradycardia in dogs. Always verify the heart rate with auscultation (do not rely on the ECG machine for the rate) and always check potassium concentration in pets with significant bradycardia "see page 81".

Tachycardia algorithm

An algorithm to follow for diagnosis and treatment of significant tachycardia in dogs. Always verify the heart rate with auscultation (do not rely on the ECG machine for the rate) "see page 82".

Asystole algorithm (CPR)

An algorithm to follow for administering cardiopulmonary resuscitation in dogs and cats. *Source: J Vet Emerg Crit Care* 2012; 22(S1): S102–131. Used with permission of Wiley "see page 83".

Arrhythmia drug chart

A list of the most commonly used drugs and currently recommended dosages for cardiac conditions in dogs and cats "see pages 84 and 85".

Life-Threatening Cardiac Emergencies for the Small Animal Practitioner, First Edition. Maureen McMichael and Ryan Fries.
© 2016 John Wiley & Sons, Inc. Published 2016 by John Wiley & Sons, Inc.

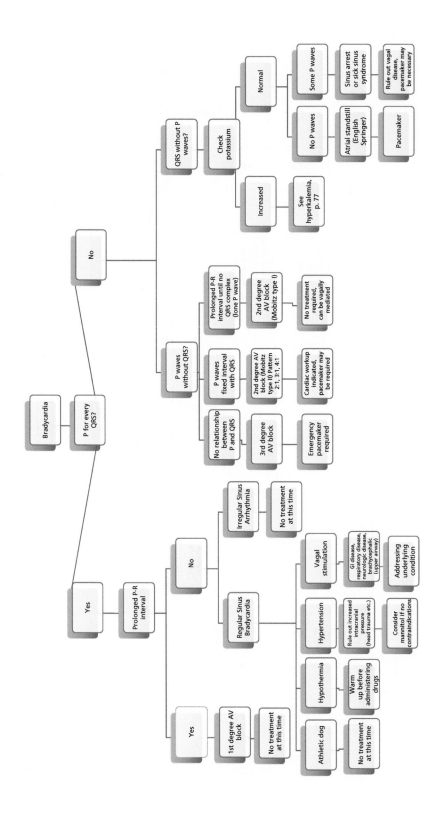

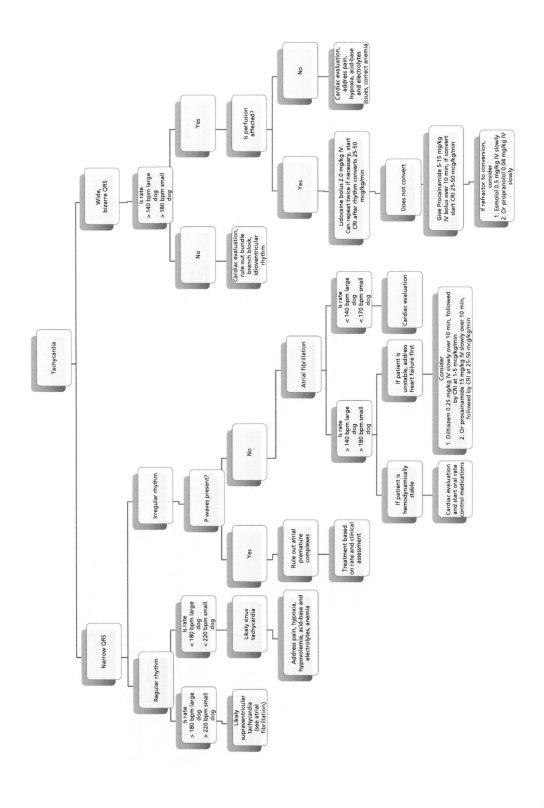

Tachycardia

Narrow QRS

Regular rhythm

- Is rate
  > 180 bpm large dog
  > 220 bpm small dog
  - Likely supraventricular tachycardia (see atrial fibrillation)

- Is rate
  < 180 bpm large dog
  < 220 bpm small dog
  - Likely sinus tachycardia
    - Address pain, hypoxia, hypovolemia, acid-base and electrolytes, anemia

Irregular rhythm

P waves present?

- Yes
  - Rule out atrial premature complexes
    - Treatment based on rate and clinical assessment

- No
  - Atrial fibrillation
    - Is rate
      > 140 bpm large dog
      > 180 bpm small dog
      - If patient is hemodynamically stable
        - Cardiac evaluation and start oral rate control medications
      - If patient is unstable, address heart failure first
        - Consider
          1. Diltiazem 0.25 mg/kg IV slowly over 10 min, followed by CRI at 1-5 mcg/kg/min
          2. Or procainamide 15 mg/kg IV slowly over 10 min, followed by CRI at 25-50 mcg/kg/min
    - Is rate
      < 140 bpm large dog
      < 170 bpm small dog
      - Cardiac evaluation

Wide, bizarre QRS

- Is rate
  > 140 bpm large dog
  > 180 bpm small dog
  - No
    - Cardiac evaluation, rule out bundle branch block, idioventricular rhythm
  - Yes
    - Is perfusion affected?
      - Yes
        - Lidocaine bolus 2.0 mg/kg IV. Can repeat twice if necessary, start CRI after rhythm converts 25-50 mcg/kg/min
          - Does not convert
            - Give Procainamide 5-15 mg/kg IV bolus over 10 min, if convert start CRI 25-50 mcg/kg/min
              - If refractor to conversion, consider
                1. Esmolol 0.5 mg/kg IV slowly
                2. Or propranolol 0.04 mg/kg IV slowly
      - No
        - Cardiac evaluation, address pain, hypoxia, acid-base and electrolytes issues, correct anemia

CPR Algorithm

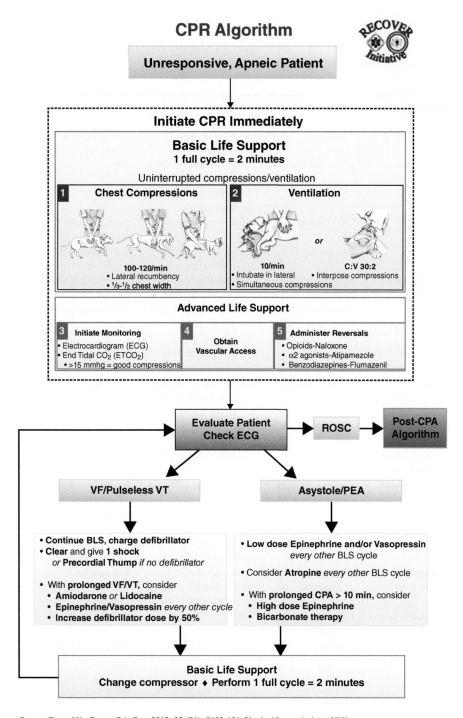

Unresponsive, Apneic Patient

Initiate CPR Immediately

Basic Life Support
1 full cycle = 2 minutes

Uninterrupted compressions/ventilation

1 Chest Compressions

100-120/min
• Lateral recumbency
• $^1/_3$-$^1/_2$ chest width

2 Ventilation

or

10/min   **C:V 30:2**
• Intubate in lateral   • Interpose compressions
• Simultaneous compressions

Advanced Life Support

3 Initiate Monitoring
• Electrocardiogram (ECG)
• End Tidal CO_2 (ETCO$_2$)
  • >15 mmhg = good compressions

4 Obtain Vascular Access

5 Administer Reversals
• Opioids-Naloxone
• α2 agonists-Atipamezole
• Benzodiazepines-Flumazenil

Evaluate Patient Check ECG → **ROSC** → **Post-CPA Algorithm**

VF/Pulseless VT

• **Continue BLS, charge defibrillator**
• **Clear** and give **1 shock**
  or **Precordial Thump** *if no defibrillator*

• With **prolonged VF/VT,** consider
  • **Amiodarone** *or* **Lidocaine**
  • **Epinephrine/Vasopressin** *every other cycle*
  • **Increase defibrillator dose by 50%**

Asystole/PEA

• **Low dose Epinephrine and/or Vasopressin**
  every other BLS cycle

• Consider **Atropine** *every other* BLS cycle

• With **prolonged CPA > 10 min,** consider
  • **High dose Epinephrine**
  • **Bicarbonate therapy**

Basic Life Support
Change compressor ♦ Perform 1 full cycle = 2 minutes

Source: From *J Vet Emerg Crit Care* 2012; 22 (S1): S102-131. Used with permission of Wiley.

Arrhythmia Drug Chart

A list of the most commonly used drugs and currently recommended dosages for cardiac conditions in dogs and cats.

DRUG	Mechanism	K9 dose	Feline dose
Acetylsalicylic acid (aspirin)	Antiplatelet	1.0 mg/kg PO q24h (low dose)	1.0 mg/kg PO q24h (low dose)
Amiodarone	Antiarrhythmic	10–20 mg/kg PO q24h for 7–10 days then reduce to 3–15 mg/kg q24h	NA
Amlodipine	Ca⁺⁺ channel blocker	0.06–1 mg/kg PO q24h	0.1–0.25 mg/kg PO q24h
Atenolol	Beta blocker	0.25–1.0 mg/kg PO q24h–q12h	6–12.5 mg/cat PO q24h–q12h
Atropine sulfate	Parasympatholytic	0.04 mg/kg IV, IM, SC	0.04 mg/kg IV, IM, SC
Butorphanol	Analgesic	0.2–0.4 mg/kg IV	0.1–0.4 mg/kg IV
L-Carnitine	Amino acid for DCM	50–100 mg/kg PO q8h	50–100 mg/kg q24h
Carvedilol	Alpha, beta blocker	0.1–1 mg/kg PO q24h–q12h	NA
Clopidogrel	Antiplatelet	1–2 mg/kg PO q12h	18.75 mg/cat PO q24h
Digoxin	Positive inotrope	0.005 mg/kg PO q12h, max dose 0.25 mg q12h	0.03 mg/cat ¼ of a 0.125 mg tab PO q48h
Diltiazem a. Cardizem (non-sustained) b. Dilacor XR (60 mg tablets inside capsule) c. Cardizem CD	Ca⁺⁺ channel blocker	0.05–0.25 mg/kg slow IV over 10 min a. 0.5–1.3 mg/kg PO q8h b. 2–4 mg/kg PO q12h	a. 7.5 mg/cat PO q12h–8h b. 30–60 mg/cat q24–12h c. 10 mg/kg PO q24h
Dobutamine	Positive inotrope	2–20 µg/kg/min IV CRI in D5W	2–10 µg/kg/min Toxicity likely in cats
Dopamine	Vasopressor	2–8 µg/kg/min	2–8 µg/kg/min
Enalapril	ACE inhibitor	0.5 mg/kg PO q24h–q12h	0.25–0.5 mg/kg PO q24h
Enoxaparin (Lovenox)	Low molecular weight heparin	NA	0.75 mg/kg SC q6h
Epinephrine	Vasopressor used for cardiac arrest, anaphylaxis	0.01–0.1 mg/kg IV	0.01–0.1 mg/kg IV
Esmolol	Beta blocker—rapid onset	50–100 µg/kg/min IV CRI Do not use with CHF/ bradycardia	NA

DRUG	Mechanism	K9 dose	Feline dose
Dalteparin (Fragmin)	Low molecular weight heparin	150 U/kg SC q6–8h	150 U/kg q6–8h
Furosemide	Loop diuretic	2–4 mg/kg IV, IM q1–6h as needed or 1–2 mg/kg/h CRI until RR halved	2–4 mg/kg IV, IM q8–12h or 0.5–1 mg/kg/h CRI until RR halved
Heparin	Anticoagulant	150–300 U/kg SC q6–8h	150–200 U/kg SC q8h
Isoproterenol	Beta agonist	0.1–2 µg/kg/min IV CRI to effect	0.1–2 µg/kg/min IV CRI to effect
Lidocaine	Na channel blocker	2–4 mg/kg IV then 25–75 µg/kg/min CRI	**Caution!** Toxic in cats at higher doses. Use 1/10 dog dose 0.2–0.4 mg/kg IV
Magnesium sulfate	For ventricular arrhythmias	0.15–0.3 mEq/kg Slow IV	0.15–0.3 mEq/kg Slow IV
Methadone	Analgesia	0.1–0.2 mg/kg IV	0.1–0.2 mg/kg IV
Mexiletine	Antiarrhythmic	4–8 mg/kg PO q8–q12h	NA
Nitroglycerin 2% ointment	Transdermal venodilator	1/4 to 2-inch strip q6–8h apply to skin	1/8–1/4-inch strip q8h apply to skin
Nitroprusside	Vasodilator Monitor BP, hypotension likely at higher doses **DO NOT FLUSH** Can be fatal	0.5–10 µg/kg/min, increase by 0.5 µg/kg/min q15min until dyspnea lessens/ hypotension occurs	0.5–10 µg/kg/min, increase by 0.5 µg/kg/min q15min until dyspnea lessens/ hypotension occurs
Pimobendan	Positive inotrope, vasodilator	0.25–0.35 mg/kg PO q12h on empty stomach	1.25–2.5 mg/cat PO q8h
Procainamide	Antiarrhythmic	5–25 mg/kg IV slow (10 min) 25–50 µg/kg/min	1–2 mg/kg IV slow 10–20 µg/kg/min
Propranolol	Beta blocker	0.5–1.0 mg/kg PO q8h	2.5–10 mg/cat PO q12–8h
Sildenafil	Phosphodiesterase inhibitor	1–3 mg/kg PO q12–8h	NA
Sotolol	Antiarrhythmic	0.5–2.0 mg/kg PO q12h	10–40 mg/cat PO q12h
Spironolactone	Potassium-sparing diuretic	1–2 mg/kg PO q12–24h	1–2 mg/kg PO q12–24h
Taurine	Amino acid for DCM	500–1000 mg/dog PO q12h	250–500 mg/cat PO q12h
Warfarin	Anticoagulant	0.1–0.2 mg/kg PO q24h	0.2–0.5 mg/cat PO q24h

Further reading

1 Ettinger SJ, Felman EC. *Textbook of Veterinary Internal Medicine*, 7th edn, 2010.
2 Cote E, MacDonald KA, Meurs KM. *Feline Cardiology*, 1st edn, 2011.
3 Tilley LP. *Essentials of Canine and Feline Electrocardiography: Interpretation and Treatment*, 3rd edn, 1992.
4 Fox PR, Sisson D, Moise NS. *Textbook of Canine and Feline Cardiology*, 1999.
5 Kittleson MD, Kienle RD. *Small Animal Cardiovascular Medicine*, 1998.
6 Gordon SG, Estrade AH. *The ABCDs of Small Animal Cardiology: A Practical Manual*, 2013.
7 Boon J. *Two-Dimensional and M-Mode Echocardiography for the Small Animal Practitioner*, 2nd edn, 2016.

Life-Threatening Cardiac Emergencies for the Small Animal Practitioner, First Edition. Maureen McMichael and Ryan Fries.
© 2016 John Wiley & Sons, Inc. Published 2016 by John Wiley & Sons, Inc.

Index

Life-Threatening Cardiac Emergencies for the Small Animal Practitioner, First Edition. Maureen McMichael and Ryan Fries.
© 2016 John Wiley & Sons, Inc. Published 2016 by John Wiley & Sons, Inc.

Printed and bound by CPI Group (UK) Ltd, Croydon, CR0 4YY

27/10/2024

14580247-0001